CREATING JOY AND MEANING FOR THE DEMENTIA PATIENT

CREATING JOY AND MEANING FOR THE DEMENTIA PATIENT

A Caregiver's Guide to Connection and Hope

Ronda Parsons

ROWMAN & LITTLEFIELD
Lanham • Boulder • New York • London

Published by Rowman & Littlefield
A wholly owned subsidiary of The Rowman & Littlefield Publishing Group,
Inc.
4501 Forbes Boulevard, Suite 200, Lanham, Maryland 20706
www.rowman.com

Unit A, Whitacre Mews, 26-34 Stannary Street, London SE11 4AB

British Library Cataloguing in Publication Information Available

Library of Congress Cataloging-in-Publication Data

Parsons, Ronda.
Creating joy and meaning for the dementia patient : a caregiver's guide to connection and hope /
Ronda Parsons.
pages cm
ISBN 978-1-4422-2755-2 (cloth : alk. paper) -- ISBN 978-1-4422-2756-9 (electronic)
1. Dementia--Patients--Care--Psychological aspects. 2. Dementia--Nursing. 3. Caregivers. I. Title.
RC521.P38 2014
616.8'3--dc23
2014042665

∞™ The paper used in this publication meets the minimum requirements of
American National Standard for Information Sciences Permanence of Paper
for Printed Library Materials, ANSI/NISO Z39.48-1992.

Printed in the United States of America

To Nan Alice, my partner on a journey neither of us would have chosen, but one filled with countless miracles all the same.

To Jack and Marjorie, for answered prayers.

To Harry, for every single blessing.

"Sing the song of the moment . . ."

—Rabindranath Tagore

Sing the song of the moment in careless carols, in the transient light of the day;
Sing of the fleeting smiles that vanish and never look back;
Sing of the flowers that bloom and fade without regret.
Weave not in memory's thread the days that would glide into nights.
To the guests that must go bid God-speed and wipe away all traces of their
steps.
Let the moments end in moments with their cargo of fugitive songs.

With both hands snap the fetters you made with your own heart chords;
Take to your breast with a smile what is easy and simple and near.
Today is the festival of phantoms that know not when they die.
Let your laughter flush in meaningless mirth like twinkles of light on the
ripples;
Let your life lightly dance on the verge of Time like a dew on the tip of a leaf.
Strike in the chords of your harp the fitful murmurs of moments.

Rabindranath N. Tagore, "Sing the song of the moment . . .,"
Poetry, A Magazine of Verse 2, no. 3 (June 1913)

CONTENTS

ACKNOWLEDGMENTS

Appreciation is a wonderful thing. It makes what is excellent in others belong to us as well.

—Voltaire

I would like to thank my agent, Anne G. Devlin of the Max Gartenberg Literary Agency, for believing that my story was worth sharing with the world. You made a lifelong dream come true. My deepest gratitude goes to Suzanne Staszak-Silva, executive editor at Rowman and Littlefield Publishing, for her advice, expertise, and encouragement. I offer special thanks to associate editor Laura Reiter and everyone involved in the publication of this book. I would like to express my gratitude to friend and writer Imelda Cummins-DeMelkon, whose support and wisdom were invaluable during the writing of this book. I want to thank Maureen Antonelli, who always urged me to put pen to paper. I would like to offer my personal thanks to Rusty Carter of the *Virginia Gazette* for publishing my essays and being so supportive. I offer a special thanks to Harry, whose encouragement and spirit are alive between every line on these pages. I am especially grateful to my teachers and the doctors, nurses, and aides who have cared for Nan so tenderly throughout the years. You taught me how to fill her days with joy. And finally, I would like to express my deepest gratitude to the multitude of fellow caregivers that I have met along my journey. Your friendship, comradery, and support truly made all the difference.

PROLOGUE

The Turning Point

Life is a series of natural and spontaneous changes. Don't resist them; that only creates sorrow. Let reality be reality. Let things flow naturally forward in whatever way they like.

—Lao Tsu
The Complete Works of Lao Tsu

Sometimes in life when you least expect it, fate knocks at your door. You can draw your curtains, look through the peephole, and even pretend that you're not at home. But in the end, your efforts are to no avail. Fate is standing on your doorstep, tapping his toe, waiting to look you square in the eye and hand you an enormous challenge, a burden greater than any you could have imagined and certainly one you could never have predicted. In the end all you can do is swing the door wide open, stand back, take a deep breath, and face the challenge head-on. This is what happened to me in 2003 when I became responsible for the care of my mother-in-law, Nan.

Years earlier if you had told me that one day I would be managing the life of someone suffering from severe dementia, I would have said that it was impossible, out of the question. In the first place I never could have imagined myself in that role, let alone envisioned Nan spiraling down through the stages of this devastating disease. I never could have predicted that I would be forced to maneuver my way through the sibling rivalries and ancient jealousies of my husband's family. I never could have predicted that I would be called upon to provide essential care to a member of the family that I had joined through marriage. And I never could have predicted on that fateful day when I finally agreed to embrace this challenge, that I was about to embark on a journey filled with moments of all-consuming heartbreak, and surprising moments of unexpected love and joy.

Nan began showing symptoms of the early stages of dementia in 1998 when she was seventy-seven years old, but managed to live on her own for several more years with the help of nearby family and friends. However, as her disease progressed, there came a time when her behavior could no longer be overlooked or swept under the rug. Once it became obvious to her entire family that it was no longer safe for her to live alone, a debate began regarding where she would live and who would be responsible for her care.

This was an emotionally charged time for everyone involved, and it was only after countless phone calls and lengthy negotiations that a decision was reached. Nan would move to Virginia and my husband and I would be responsible for her financial and physical well-being. Through the clarity of hindsight, I realize that I was the only person who knew exactly what this meant. For although my husband loves his mother as much as any son can, the demands of his job do not allow time for the day-to-day challenges of caring for a dementia patient. I think I was the only one who fully understood that Nan's care was destined to land squarely on my shoulders.

Now if at this point in my story, I told you in a saintly and condescending voice that I welcomed this challenge and thought that it was a grand idea that Nan move into an assisted living facility near us, I fear that you would shut this book and shout "LIAR" at the top of your lungs. No, I must admit that initially I was dumbfounded and a bit angry. I had just lost my mother after a long battle with cancer and, frankly, I wasn't excited about facing another sad and draining healthcare situation.

My reluctance to take on this responsibility had nothing to do with my feelings for Nan. My affection for her runs deep, and I consider her to be an ideal mother-in-law. From the first time that we met she welcomed me with open arms and treated me with the same kindness and respect she lavished on her children. Over the years as our friendship grew, we had many wonderful and funny adventures together.

There was the Christmas Day turkey crisis of 1983, when a discrete hole in a turkey roaster made such a mess in my first kitchen that I would not be surprised if lurking somewhere deep beneath the floor boards in that old house there remains a small puddle of dried giblet grease. There was the time we decided to spend an entire weekend cutting out wood tulips on a band saw, trying to copy flowers that she had seen in a local shop. On another occasion we became so lost while trying to find an antique shop in downtown Columbus that we gave up on our treasure hunt, only to stumble on a diner that made delicious ice cream churned the old-fashioned way.

No, she and I are great friends, which only made my hesitation more heart wrenching. And it is also why, through gritted teeth, I agreed that it would be best if Nan moved near us in Virginia. Little did I know then that she and I were beginning on a journey filled with great highs and deep sorrows—one I could never have imagined, one that changed who I am today, and oddly, one that I would not have missed for the world.

We are taught from an early age to always try to *do the right thing*. In today's world of slogans, catchphrases, and five-second sound bites, it seems to make perfect sense, another item checked off our list. But in reality when faced with the heartbreaking challenge of caring for a dementia patient day-in and day-out for years on end, it is no longer a cliché. It is a demanding reality that can bring the most loving caregiver to their emotional breaking point. For dementia does not just affect the sufferer; it reaches its tentacles into the lives that orbit around the patient, often leaving those lives exhausted and defeated.

When I first began caring for Nan I operated in a defensive mode, solving problems as they were thrown at me. I would lay awake at night trying to fix unfixable problems and searching for answers that did not exist. I made lists and attacked daily problems with vigor, but in the end I always felt taxed and frustrated. The sad truth was that despite all my efforts, Nan was drifting further into oblivion each day and I was finding it increasingly difficult to reach her mentally and emotionally. At one point her behavior became so disruptive that her doctors suggested that she begin taking a series of drugs to keep her calm. Although I knew that this would probably be necessary at some time in the future, I wasn't ready to throw in the towel just yet. I was frustrated, but not defeated.

One afternoon as I was driving home from yet another exasperating visit, feeling limp with worry and defeat, I had an epiphany that changed everything. I guess you could call it my aha moment, my turning point. If I was going to survive I would have to change my attitude and find ways for Nan and me to forge some kind of a meaningful channel of communication. She wasn't happy and neither was I.

Up until this point I had taken my cues from her, spending all my energy begging her to cooperate. Every day I found myself pleading with her to take her medicine, eat lunch, change her clothes, and take a shower. I needed a new approach, a new strategy. I had to find a way to take charge of the situation. Since I was in this battle for the long haul, I had best buck up and try a new approach.

Through observation I had come to realize that Nan no longer lived in a world made up of days or even hours, but instead she lived inside spontaneous flashes of reality, like fireflies that flicker in the night sky. In other words, Nan was living her life from moment to moment. As quickly as recognition arrived, it was gone again. I knew instinctively that although her understanding was temporary, these moments were not unimportant. Over time I came to learn that no happiness is too small or its effect too insignificant to affect positive change. For when she is content and at peace, the old Nan from long ago would suddenly appear out of nowhere in the guise of a familiar comment or facial expression. Then like quicksilver she would vanish. But those momentary associations were all the encouragement I needed to keep trying to build a bridge and forge a connection between us. Those moments reminded me of the woman I missed so terribly and proved to me that she was still in there, lost in dementia's thick fog. It was then that I made it my mission to harness Nan's moments and effectively utilize their power in order to bring joy and meaning into her life.

I started small. At first my goal was just to see her smile and react positively to a brief interaction or to an activity that we did together. I brought favorite foods for her to eat. I played CDs of the old Baptist hymns she loved to sing. We fed birds as we sat outside in her courtyard. I tried to create little surprises for her that would trigger even the briefest moment of happiness. Granted, I wasn't always successful. It took time for me to figure out her triggers. But slowly my small successes began to build and it wasn't long before those difficult days began to become easier for each of us to bear.

We sat in rocking chairs, smelled flowers, and watched birds. We browsed through old family photographs. We sang songs and listened to her favorite music. Occasionally we even danced together. Yes, I discovered that it is possible to jitterbug in a wheelchair. We ate chocolate ice cream, painted her fingernails, and scented her room. We prayed and talked about the many blessings in our lives. I recounted stories that reminded her that she was a wonderful person who had led an extraordinary life.

By the end of the first year, I had found so many ways to connect with Nan, that I began writing them down in a journal I called my *Ideas Book*. As the pages filled, so did my contentment as a caregiver. I found that as my attitude relaxed and calmed, so did Nan's. I learned that as a caregiver, I possessed the power to alter the tempo and undercurrent of our relationship. I could choose to inject hope and understanding into this heartbreaking situation. Somehow in all the madness, as I tackled the problems that plague all dementia patients, I was able to find shared moments of sweet happiness. It was nothing short of a miracle.

I know that this may all sound too good to be true. Understand that I am not saying that Nan and I never had difficulties again, or that she suddenly became a rational and whole human being. No, I am not saying that at all. But I am asking you to rethink your strategy. Instead of letting an endless stream of daily problems consume your time together, rethink your priorities. Rethink how you can inject small moments of joy and happiness into the life of your loved one. Rethink the attitude you bring to your visits. Rethink the power you possess to make things better. Rethink your role as a caregiver. Stand back. Take another picture.

Little did I know at the time, but experts in the field of dementia were in agreement with my approach to Nan's care. The plan that I developed naturally through intuition is in fact in alignment with methods that are being implemented in both the United States and Europe. This knowledge gives me hope—hope that families will begin to celebrate what a dementia patient can bring to their lives, rather than see them as an inconvenience to be relegated to the sidelines. It gives me hope that others are also embracing the concept that under certain circumstances, it is best to focus on the quality of our days, rather than the quantity. And mostly, it validates my approach and the likelihood that I am bringing joy and meaning into Nan's life.

I am particularly inspired by Thomas Kitwood's 1997 groundbreaking work entitled *Dementia Reconsidered: The Person Comes First* in which he advocates a new "person-centered" care for dementia patients. He encourages us "to return to aspects of our being that are much older in evolutionary terms: more in tune with the body and its functions, closer to the life of instinct."[1]

Sometimes I catch my breath when I think of how different my life would be if I had not learned from my frustrations and found my way to the activities detailed in this book. My relationship with Nan would be very different. I could have very easily missed out on one of the most profound experiences of my life. The time that I have spent with Nan has become sacred to me, filled with unexpected wonders and many beautiful and funny surprises. Oddly, she has buoyed me as much as I have helped her, and together we have been able to find our way, in the dark at times, but always managing to stay the course.

This is not a technical manual about dementia and Alzheimer's disease. I'll leave the neurological changes and drug therapies to the experts. No, this is a book about the person that still lives inside each dementia patient and specific activities that allow them to once again experience the beauty of being alive. To give this gift to someone you love is a blessing beyond words and a joy indescribable.

I know that these strategies work. I have witnessed pure joy on Nan's face as we turned the pages of her *Memory Book* or ate a strawberry right off the vine. As caregivers, we have the ability to set the tone of the relationship.

And here is another detail that cannot be overstated. While I was creating moments of peace and joy for Nan, I could not help but spill a little happiness onto myself.

Today Nan's disease has progressed to the point that it is necessary for her to live in a nursing facility. Oftentimes when I come to visit I look around at all the individuals suffering from dementia or Alzheimer's disease and I wish I could meet each one of them as they used to be long before disease ravaged their minds. Doctors. Lawyers. Teachers. Mothers. Even if only for fifteen short minutes, I would love to know who they were: their personalities, their senses of humor, their essence. I'd like to be able to tell them how deeply their lives have touched mine and that I am forever changed for having known them.

But most of all I'd like to talk to Nan again. The real Nan. The intelligent funny woman I remember her to be. Ten years of conversation in only fifteen minutes? Do you think I could manage it? Maybe not, but oh, how I'd love to try.

I

GRABBING AT SHADOWS

I think that wherever your journey takes you, there are new gods waiting there, with divine patience—and laughter.

—Susan M. Watkins

Not many people can say that the movie *Sleepless in Seattle* changed their life. In fact, I might be the only person. Never could I have imagined that this charming romantic film would set in motion a chain of events that would impact my life for the next fifteen years. The aftermath would rock my husband's family to its foundation and send ripples through all our lives like a stone dropped into a still pond.

On a beautiful autumn afternoon in 1998, Nan and I went to see the movie *Sleepless in Seattle* at the local Cineplex near our home in Virginia. She was visiting us from Ohio to escape the first snows of winter, which at the age of seventy-seven were becoming difficult for her to endure. She also needed a change of scenery. For the past few months when we spoke on the telephone, her mood had seemed sad and distant. Although her husband had passed away five years earlier, she never really seemed to have moved forward. Her grief had remained fresh and trapped just beneath the surface of everything in her daily life.

From the first time we met, Nan and I were great friends. We never engaged in those tiresome in-law turf wars that you hear so much about. No, she had immediately opened her heart to me and I in turn respected her for raising the man who was going to share my life. I am always baffled by daughters-in-law who constantly complain about their husband's mother. Nan created and formed the person I love above anyone else in the world. In my opinion this deserves a bit of respect.

Whenever she came to visit I made a special effort to plan activities that she seldom took time for in Ohio. We would eat at a favorite lunch spot, go shopping, visit an art museum, or attend a play. And sometimes, like on this particular autumn day, we would forgo a healthy lunch and eat hot, buttered popcorn in the darkness of an afternoon matinee.

When the lights came up at the end of the movie and the audience was still whispering about the final romantic scene, I looked over at Nan and asked, "How did you like it?" She replied, "It was fine." This seemed odd, so I kept probing. "Wasn't Jonah adorable? And didn't you just love the part when Annie was having dinner with Walter and looked out at the Empire State Building and realized that she just had to go and see if Sam was waiting for her?" To which she replied, "What? Oh, yeah. That was cute." Cute? There was nothing cute about it. This bizarre response was coming from a woman who was a complete pushover when it came to anything involving romance, holidays, and adorable children. Something wasn't adding up.

As we walked back to the car my questions became broader. I asked her which part of the movie she liked best and whether she had predicted that Sam and Annie would end up together. Her responses were curt and gruff. As I drove home in the evening twilight I decided that either she couldn't remember the movie or she was unable to follow the plot. Either way, something was terribly wrong.

When I first met my in-laws they lived deep in the flat farmlands of central Ohio, in an old white farmhouse bordered on each side by corn and soybean fields. It was perfectly situated. Behind the back porch and flapping clothesline stood two large barns as white as the puffy clouds that fill the endless Midwest skies. To the right of the house, surrounded by ancient apple trees and wild honeysuckle, was an enormous garden rototilled and planted with vegetables destined for autumn canning.

This was a working farm run by working people who had never held a mortgage or applied for a credit card. They paid cash for what they needed and believed in saving for the inevitable rainy day. A tough industrious couple who knew how to scrimp, save, and *make do*. They loved country life and trusted in the mercy of God.

Born in 1921, Nan's character was molded by two monumental life events: the austerity of the Great Depression and her mother's sudden death on her eighth birthday. I don't think she ever completely recovered from the devastation of losing her mother so young, for she continued to speak of it long after dementia had ravaged her mind. She carried it through life like a stone rattling in a tin bucket.

After her mother's burial, Nan, her brother, and two sisters were packed up and sent by train to stay with relatives in Winston-Salem, North Carolina. I am not sure how long they were away from their father and everything that was familiar in their lives. Nan's recollection of these events made it seem like she was gone for years, but it may have just seemed that way to her. I have to remember that although a grown woman was telling me this story, she was still viewing these events through the eyes of a small child. It was during this time that Nan, as the oldest girl, became mother, teacher, and protector of her three siblings. She proudly bore this role and never completely relinquished it.

When her father finally summoned his four children home to Ohio, they were greeted by their new stepmother, Faye, a disagreeable woman straight out of the pages of *Cinderella*. The years that followed were incredibly hard and difficult, but much to Nan's credit, they all thrived. Her means of escape was a failed first marriage and the outbreak of World War II when she decided to enlist in the WAVES.

It speaks to Nan's character that years later, when Faye was very old and had no one to care for her, she offered her a home at the farm. Although the gesture was motivated by her love for her father, she meant every word of her offer. Had a distant relative not stepped in, I am certain that Nan would have been true to her word and provided a safe haven for the stepmother who had made her childhood so difficult.

Nan was half magpie and half saint, a wonderfully quirky personality combination that you rarely meet today. Like so many others who were raised during the harsh years of the Depression, she was a collector of things, anything she found beautiful or possessing sentimental meaning. When she wasn't collecting, she was dispensing kindness by the bushel, living a selfless life built on the resolve that bad luck will turn into good and decency lives inside each of us. Having grown up in a family whose unspoken motto was, *If mama ain't happy, ain't nobody happy,* I found this attitude intriguing and refreshing, like a cool drink of water on a hot summer's day.

Nan's farmhouse was her nest and like a magpie she filled it to the brim with the treasures of a lifetime. Occasionally she'd splurged on something new that caught her eye, but more often than not her treasures were gifts she had received or items left behind by relatives that had passed on. It didn't matter to her how much they cost or if they matched her décor; like a bird collecting shiny objects, she tended and cared for them equally. The lunch pail that Great-Uncle Millard carried into the coal mines of West Virginia sat on the hearth. Hand embroidered pillowcases and lace linens once belonging to a distant cousin dressed the beds. A quilt pieced from 1930s trouser samples was draped over the sofa. Trinkets her children had bought or won for her at the Licking County Fair were proudly displayed. The soft pink and gray china she earned by saving 1960s gasoline credits held a place of prominence in her dining room hutch. She was a collector of memories, the memory keeper, the guardian of her loved one's labors and past dreams.

Years later when her husband had passed on and she could no longer stay at the farm, we all gathered to sort and disperse her belongings. I was touched to find tucked in the back of a drawer letters that I had written to her when I first began dating her son. They had been bundled with a piece of saved kitchen twine and tied with a shoelace bow.

In the late 1960s the Parsonses bought a small general store in the village of Homer and Nan became the proprietress of Homer Market. When my then boyfriend took me there for the first time, I felt like I had disembarked from the Cannonball in Petticoat Junction and was standing in front of Sam Drucker's market. It was an honest-to-goodness general store, with wood plank floors and enormous high ceilings, where you could browse through everything from canned goods and brooms to freshly butchered meats. It was the town hub because it faced State Route 661 that ran right through the center of the village. Its long front porch was perfect for the long-ago pastimes of watching neighbors and counting cars.

To this day, long after the store has been abandoned, we honk and salute the old market building anytime we are passing through. We do this in honor of Nan and those bygone days when a small market in a small town was able to survive and when neighbors would stop in just to buy a cold pop cooled in an enormous Pepsi soda chest, the kind with a chrome bottle opener built right into the side. As I sit and write this, the old metal *Homer Market* sign complete with Pepsi logo is sitting on a shelf in my garage, rusty and a bit dented at the corners where it was once nailed to the white planked wood on the side of that old market building.

Even though the town encompassed only a few small blocks, it managed to squeeze in a post office, library, elementary school, a few small houses, and of course a church. Homer Market was Nan's gift to the town. I don't think she ever really made a profit; she was too busy giving away as much food as she sold. No one in Homer went hungry as long as Nan owned her store.

All these thoughts and many more swirled through my mind as we drove home from the movie that evening. I could tell by her curt and almost angry responses that she was well aware of her confusion. It wasn't until later that I learned just how easy it is for an individual in the early stages of dementia to bluff their way through conversations and interactions with family members. Only when pressed for concrete answers to specific questions are they no longer able to fake it. I wondered how long this had been going on. I decided not to say anything else that evening but to talk to my husband and his sister as soon as possible. If she became this upset just being asked about a movie, I could not imagine what her response would be if I suggested that she might be losing her memory.

Looking back I can plainly see that there had been signs of a problem long before the afternoon she and I went to the movies. Actually, when the three of us compared notes our discoveries were quite alarming. Her innate intelligence had tricked us. She was able to hide her difficulties for so long because she communicated so beautifully on the telephone. Easy answers to everyday questions rolled off her tongue, and as long as the subject matter remained light and general she knew by rote how to respond appropriately. You only noticed that her mental capabilities were slipping if you spent an extended period of time with her and observed her as she went about her daily activities.

A year earlier in September of 1997 when she was seventy-six years old, Nan began having symptoms of a heart attack while she was having her hair shampooed and set at the local Chatter and Curl. The chances of an ambulance arriving quickly deep in the remote countryside is a real gamble. So when Nan started feeling sick the owner dropped everything, closed the shop and sped her to the nearest hospital. Within hours she had suffered a massive heart attack, died, and was revived with the "paddles of life." Soon after being saved she suffered a major, debilitating stroke.

All this happened on the weekend that Diana, Princess of Wales, died. The heartbreaking, dawn-to-dusk news coverage playing on the television in the hospital waiting room matched our mood. It was as if the entire world was grieving with us.

Nan endured months of physical and occupational therapy at a rehabilitation center at The Ohio State University. She may have given up and never regained her physical mobility if it had not been for her daughter. Cindi was a tireless cheerleader, visiting every day, boosting her mother's morale and encouraging her to stay focused. Although Nan never was able to move back to the farm or drive a car again, she did regain the ability to walk and care for herself independently. She went straight from the rehabilitation center to a small apartment in a retirement community in Columbus.

Nan's dementia began the following year. Neurologists believe that it was most likely caused by her massive stroke, although no one can be certain. For that matter, tests have been unable to technically determine if she is suffering from Alzheimer's disease or acute dementia. Since there is little variation in treatment, we decided not to put her through the stress of additional testing. The problem was the same regardless of what her affliction was called. After all, what was in a name? Nan's younger sister has begun displaying early onset symptoms, so her disease could have a hereditary component. We will never be completely sure because it is Nan's good fortune to have lived longer than any of her relatives in recent memory.

When the early stages of dementia begin to present themselves it is a particularly devastating time for the patient and their family. Because symptoms can be so subtle and seem to appear and then vanish, family members often underestimate the severity of the problem. After all, they look the same don't they? There is no visible sign of their disease. And to make matters more confusing, there are times when they are perfectly rational and able to function beautifully. This feeds into a family's collective wishful thinking that none of this is really happening. They tell themselves, "We are overreacting. It is just a bad day. Soon things will be back to normal. Maybe this is just a rough patch. They are getting older after all."

Driven by fear, the patient and their family create a kind of grand illusion that in the final analysis only wastes time, creates conflicts, and delays constructive goal setting. Fear in this situation not only blocks us from reality but can place our loved one in jeopardy.

After the *Sleepless in Seattle* incident, I began watching Nan closely and noticed other worrisome behaviors. For example, when we went to a restaurant she always ordered the exact same meal and beverage that I selected. And then it dawned on me. She could no longer read and interpret a menu, which made it impossible for her to select an entrée. Yes, she still recognized words and was able to read them aloud, but she was unable to interpret, retain, and analyze the information that she read. Even going out for a simple lunch had become a stressful and shame-filled experience.

Then as if overnight, Nan's cognitive difficulties accelerated. She was no longer able to administer her own medications. A daily pill organizer seemed to solve the problem for a short time, but soon this method proved to be too complicated. Then we began noticing that she was wearing the same clothes for several days in a row. Sadly the explanation for this was simple. Since she could not remember what she had worn the day before, she was unable to determine when her clothes needed to be laundered. Around this time her mail grew into enormous piles stacked on the kitchen table in her apartment. She could not distinguish bills and important correspondence from junk mail, so she saved everything. If an attempt was made to help sort through these piles, she became extremely agitated and angry. Every small decision, ones that you and I would make in a split second, was leaving her paralyzed with confusion and uncertainty.

The magnitude and rapidity of her decline were difficult for me to watch, but for my husband it was nothing short of heartbreaking. While we were visiting Columbus in 2001, we decided to try to clear out some of the clutter that had accumulated in her apartment. We were shocked at what we found. Her drawers and cabinets were stuffed with trash and debris of every kind. It was as if she no longer took out her garbage. I guess if you can't decide what is important and what isn't, the obvious solution is to keep everything. We found money tucked in shoes and Tylenol bottles. Water leaked from baskets filled with artificial flowers. During our visit she even left the water running in her bathroom sink and flooded her apartment.

But extraordinarily even in the midst of all this chaos, she had moments, even hours, of perfect clarity. We were still able to go to restaurants and take long rides in the country. We reminisced about old times and took her to visit old friends.

And therein lies the irony. This inconsistent aspect of a patient's behavior and personality explains why it is so easy for family members to keep their feet firmly planted in a state of denial. In the early stages of dementia when their loved one is able to retain some sense of normality in their daily life, it is easy to pretend that everything is okay. You tell yourself, "All they need is a helping hand every now and then. Maybe I should hire someone to come in and help them for a few hours each morning."

Unfortunately this attitude can be cataclysmic. What if the next time instead of letting the water overflow in the bathroom, Nan had forgotten to turn off the stove? By not facing the absolute truth regarding Nan's situation, we were placing her in danger. When we first began witnessing her cognitive decline, we should have developed a plan that mapped out the future. We should have faced the fact that eventually she would require daily assistance. In the clarity of hindsight I realize that we should have moved Nan into an assisted living facility much sooner than we did. We were lucky, just plain lucky, that nothing catastrophic happened while we were afraid to face the reality of her situation.

In the 1990s when Nan first began displaying symptoms of dementia, there was very little information available for worried family members or prospective caregivers. All expert information seemed to center around a negative prognosis consisting of dismal mental and behavioral projections. The worries and fears of the caregiver, both rational and irrational, were completely overlooked. In those days we had to find solutions through trial and error and by trying to apply common sense to an extremely nonsensical situation. Consequently, all of us in Nan's family made huge mistakes, mistakes that wasted emotional energy and caused friction between us. Be careful. Two traps are waiting to ensnare you, traps that made my entire family easy prey.

First, we incorrectly believed that if Nan would only concentrate harder her short-term memory would improve. After all remembering where you put your keys or if you took your 6 p.m. medicine was just a matter of remaining alert and watching the clock, right? All three of us truly believed that Nan possessed the ability to see the problem, apply self-discipline, and make the necessary corrections. If we could just get her to focus and concentrate on what she was doing, things would improve. Each of us in our own way tried to cajole her into modifying her behavior. When this didn't work we made a succession of "To Do" and "Reminder" lists for her to follow, complete with boxes for her to check as tasks were completed. This solution was only effective for a brief period of time; before long we were right back where we started.

What I didn't understand at the time was that as Nan's memory failed, her ability to problem solve and interpret information was also steadily declining. At times I became so frustrated with her that I was convinced she was being deliberately uncooperative and that her secret goal was to drive me crazy. In a way this seemed possible because there were times when Nan appeared normal and was completely lucid. I know now that this was just a mirage and that even on her good days, she was losing mental ground. She was not trying to frustrate me. She was doing her best; her best just wasn't what it used to be.

The second and even more exasperating mistake we made was to try to reason with Nan and explain why her logic was irrational. Each of us worked hard to refute her confusion by breaking down any misunderstanding into intelligent and undeniable parts. Looking back I realize that it was absolutely ridiculous to engage in a debate with a dementia sufferer, but at the time I did not understand the realities of the disease. So I continued to give it my best shot. She would share a premise that she believed to be true and I, on rebuttal, would point out where she was wrong. I made endless coherent arguments in an attempt to prove that she wasn't seeing things clearly. I was determined to gain her concurrence and help her to see the light. Surely if it were clearly explained, she would see the error of her ways. I don't have to tell you that my efforts were a massive waste of time. In the end she always became angry and I was left weak with exasperation.

A perfect example of this occurred each evening when Nan, like so many other dementia sufferers, would ask to go home. Every day without fail, Nan would call me insisting that her apartment was not her home and that I should come and get her. It was relentless, a battle we fought sometimes twice in an evening. Because she had mild dementia when she moved to her new apartment, her new home never really became embedded into her long-term memory. Consequently, she had trouble remembering where she lived and understandably this made her very agitated and desperate to find her real home. So in an effort to apply common sense I would try to reason with her logically.

For as long as I had known Nan a large sepia picture of her mother, Lillie, had hung above her bed. I would ask her to look at the picture and agree that this was her mother. Then I would logically point out that if her mother's picture is hanging above her bed, she must be in her own apartment surrounded by her belongings. She would agree, but her understanding would only last for an instant. After just a few seconds we were right back where we started and she was pleading with me to come and take her home. I felt like a mouse running on a wheel.

What I didn't realize was that in order to be able to apply logic you must have the ability to link threads of reason. Otherwise, you just end up with a tangled ball of undecipherable information. Unfortunately, Nan had lost her ability to connect the dots. She could agree on the single reality or truth, but could not assimilate the data in order to reach a logical final conclusion. I can still hear myself trying to explain to her step-by-step, that no one had burgled her apartment and stolen her television remote control, shoes, or her money. I begged her to understand that they were just misplaced. But my efforts were always an exercise in futility. I never got through. I was wasting my time.

According to the National Alzheimer's Association, more than five million Americans suffer from dementia or Alzheimer's disease, a number that is predicted to escalate as the baby boomers continue to age. As staggering as these statistics are, they only tell half of the story. "In 2013, 15.5 million caregivers provided 17.7 billion hours of unpaid care, valued at $220 billion."[1] Typically, caregivers find themselves in a situation that they never could have imagined. The enormous emotional, physical, and financial strains that they endure cannot be over-estimated.

At least this information tells us that we are not alone. Waking up each morning faced with another day of coaxing, pleading, and physical exertion can make you feel as if you are the only person in the world with this problem. Caretaking can feel very lonely. I remember seeing others going merrily about their lives while I felt stuck like a fly that had landed on sticky paper. I'm not saying that every day was terrible. But even Nan's good days often left me feeling physically and emotionally drained. And the uncertainty of her situation only exacerbated this problem.

Like most dementia suffers, Nan's behavioral and mental changes seemed to progress in fits and starts. She had periods when her symptoms would advance in a whirl of acceleration and then they would level off for a few months, or as in one instance, a year. Then her disease would resurface and she would go through another period of decline followed by a period of calm equilibrium. This up-and-down pattern continues even to this day, although the peaks and valleys are not as extreme as they once were.

Helplessly watching someone you love slowly change and slip away is unfathomably sad and frightening. Each new symptom is like a punch in the stomach. The slowness of it only adds to your agony and increases your fear of what the future holds.

Fear is an odd and deceptive emotion, a chameleon of sorts. One minute it can appear as anger; the next, as frustration. It has a negative impact on our behavior and feelings. When fighting dementia, fear often outruns our patience and taints our common sense, leaving us to march in futile circles around the same mountain again and again. Fear stifles our compassion and constructs insurmountable walls against the truth. Fear clouds our vision, leaving us to search in the dark for answers that were in front of us all along.

In order to be effective in any sorrowful situation, we must face things as they really are, accept what we know to be true, and keep moving forward one step at a time. Don't feel defeated if you have spent too long consumed with worry for your loved one. It is never too late to work through your fears and quiet the negative voices that play in your mind. By sharing my experiences I hope to show you how to move forward in this process. I want to encourage you to offer yourself the same patience and compassion that you shower on your loved one. For it was only when I stopped being afraid of Nan's future and how it was going to impact me, that I was able to accept her prognosis and open my eyes to the many blessing still present in her life.

The National Alzheimer's Association lists the following warning signs and indicators that an individual may be suffering from the early stages of dementia or Alzheimer's disease.

- Memory loss that disrupts daily life
- Challenges in planning events or solving problems
- Difficulty completing familiar tasks at home, at work, or at leisure
- Confusion with time or place
- Trouble understanding visual images and spatial relationships
- New problems with words when speaking or writing
- Misplacing things and losing the ability to retrace steps
- Decreased and poor judgment
- Withdrawal from work or social activities
- Changes in mood or social activities[2]

By the spring of 2003, Nan's symptoms had reached a fever pitch and the severity of her symptoms could no longer be ignored. When she saw her reflection in the mirror she thought that there was another woman in the room with her. She began cursing and using foul language. She thought what she saw on television was happening right there in her presence. If she saw a program where guns were fired, she thought someone was firing a gun in her room. It became difficult for her to find her way to her apartment after the evening meal. And most disturbing of all, she began hallucinating and seeing barking dogs that were not there.

The time had come. The inevitable had happened. The prognosis had been accurate all along. Denial was no longer possible. Immediate action was necessary. She needed our support more than ever before, so it was decided that she would come and live near us in Virginia.

I admit that as an only child, I don't completely understand the notion of sibling rivalry, let alone how it carries over into relationships in adulthood. Harry has one sister, so I knew that we had a fifty-fifty chance of becoming Nan's primary caretakers. But I assumed that all things considered, Nan would move to North Carolina to be near her daughter. So even though I knew intellectually that it was possible, I actually never expected Nan to become our responsibility. It was only after his sister told me flat-out that she wasn't taking her mother that reality finally hit me in the face. We had no choice; or rather I had no choice. Nan was coming to Virginia.

At this point I must include a caveat. If I could rewrite history and change my story right here with Nan being swept off to live with her daughter in North Carolina, I wouldn't. No, I would not change one thing. Caring for Nan has taught me infinite lessons, more than could ever be squeezed into the pages of a book. I see myself in a new light. I see Nan in a new light. I see the world with new eyes.

Caring for Nan has been like grabbing at shadows, shadows that are growing long and distorted as evening draws near. The bright sun that was once directly overhead is nearing sunset—that time when shadows grow larger than the life that supports them and they seem stretched almost to their breaking point. As twilight approaches, the shadows mock me, tempting me to try to coax her back one last time. But these phantoms are just that, apparitions impossible to catch and not meant to be detained this close to nightfall.

I could never have imagined or predicted the emotional highs and lows that lay before me on my journey with Nan. I've had days of frustration, anger, and utter defeat. I've had moments so sweet that I thought my heart would break wide open, and times I've wanted to turn and walk away. But I am so thankful that I didn't. For somewhere in the middle of all this chaos, just when I least expected it, Nan and I would manage to find our way in the gathering shadows, sometimes moving just an inch, sometimes a bit further, but always moving forward in the direction of the light.

INSIGHTS

- Take notice if your loved one's reaction to a situation seems odd or out of character.
- If your loved one begins displaying any of the warning signs of dementia or Alzheimer's disease, schedule an appointment with their physician.

- When deciding who will manage your loved one's care, set aside personal differences and select an individual who is physically and mentally up for the challenge.
- Realize that a diagnosis of dementia is difficult for everyone in the patient's life. Remember that everyone processes information differently. Keep in mind that this diagnosis can be particularly difficult for a family member who has unresolved issues with the patient.
- Be aware that some verbal responses like answering simple questions can be recited from memory. Don't accept these responses as proof that your loved one does not have dementia.
- Realize that asking your loved one to concentrate or try harder will not improve their cognitive abilities.
- Avoid trying to reason with your loved one in order to gain their concurrence. Often this will just make them angry and frustrated.
- Do not argue with your loved one. Be patient and remember that they cannot control many of their feelings and actions.
- Make easy-to-read checklists for your loved one to follow. This is especially helpful in the early stages of the disease.
- Purchase single-dose medicine dispensers that are clearly labeled with the time and day of the week. Fill them in advance so that you can ensure that your loved one takes the correct doses at the correct times.
- Consider hiring a care worker to help your loved one remain organized and keep their environment safe.
- Consider managing your loved one's incoming bills and financial accounts. This will ensure that monies are not being squandered and that their bills are being paid on time.
- Program your phone number into the speed-dial of your loved one's telephone so that it is easy for them to contact you.
- Don't wait. The earlier that the disease is diagnosed, the sooner you can begin ensuring their safety and planning for their future.

2

ACCEPTANCE

Let the light of late afternoon
shine through chinks in the barn, moving
up the bales as the sun moves down. . . .

Let the dew collect on the hoe abandoned
in long grass. Let the stars appear
and the moon disclose her silver horn. . . .

Let it come, as it will, and don't
be afraid. God does not leave us
comfortless, so let evening come.

—Jane Kenyon
"Let Evening Come"

Once she had been Nan Parsons, an independent and defiantly strong woman, quick witted and filled with humor. Today if you came to visit her, you would find a quiet gentle soul seated in a Geri-Chair who seldom speaks, preferring instead to sit and hum soft impromptus. When she does communicate, although it is with her usual animated vigor, it is in a language of her own creation, in words that only she understands.

There was a time when simply pointing out the difference between these two Nans would have caused me great anxiety and sadness. But that was years ago now. No, I long ago said my goodbyes to the Nan I once knew and made my peace with her understudy, the diminutive woman who has taken her place. She looks like Nan and tries her best to act her part, but she only gets her lines right on occasion. As if illuminated by the desolate "ghost light" on an empty stage, she always delivers a lackluster performance that leaves the audience feeling cheated and aching for the return of the main attraction.

Of all the hurdles that I have faced while caring for Nan, acceptance has been my greatest challenge. Not only have I had to deal with the sadness of watching the deterioration of someone I love, but I have also had to find a way to cope with feelings of resentment that surfaced after being forced to take on this enormous responsibility.

There is an old adage that states that if you want to know how a prospective husband will treat you in marriage, you should pay close attention to how he treats his mother. On this front I won the jackpot. I have never seen a mother-child relationship with the depth of spirit and respect that exists between my husband, Harry, and his mother. For her part, she has always been his champion, eager to share her wisdom and see him succeed in the world. His needs have always come before hers. When he was young, she spread margarine on her toast so that he could have butter. She saved books of Green Stamps that she traded for his first baseball glove. And when it finally arrived she was the one who taught him how to pitch a fastball like the pros so that no batter stood a chance. In college when he was working split shifts at a glass factory, no matter what time of day, she always had a hot meal prepared so that he never went to work or bed hungry. Nan is proud of her boy and often tells me how similar their personalities are. When it comes to her son, her pride is impossible to hide.

My husband learned how to live his life by how his mother conducted herself in the world. He learned empathy from her tenderness. He learned wisdom from her patience. He learned gratitude from her humility. He learned love from her tender spirit. And in return, he strives each day to pay back each of her selfless acts of kindness with his respect, love, and devotion.

Families are complicated units, entities with their own histories and rules governing how they function. They have pasts so complex and tangled, that an outsider has no hope of ever completely unwinding the string back to the original point where it first became knotted. Even those within a family are often bewildered as to why they operate as they do. For this reason, I will never know the exact *why* of how I came to care for Nan. I can only tell the story as it unfolded, from the vantage point of someone who was not born into the Parsons family.

When it finally became obvious that Nan needed to move into an assisted living facility, Harry and his sister had two options. Nan could leave Ohio and move to North Carolina to be near her daughter, or she could come to Virginia and live near my husband and me. As I have mentioned before, my first choice was to have her move near her daughter. I thought that my sister-in-law would prefer having her mother close to her. In my mind it was only natural. In the end, however, my sister-in-law, who had lived near her mother for years, rejected this idea and insisted that my husband and I become responsible for Nan's care. If I told you that I thought this was fair, I would be lying. I had never heard of an in-law taking on this kind of responsibility. To this day whenever Nan and I meet someone new, they always assume that Nan is my mother. After I explain that I am in fact her daughter-in-law, people are often shocked and a bit surprised. Although I still disagree with my sister-in-law's decision, over time I became grateful for her stance and my many precious years with Nan.

When all this was taking place I had technically lived in Williamsburg for a few years, but emotionally I was still just getting acquainted. Because my mother was ill, I had spent the last eighteen months of my mother's life shuttling between my home in Williamsburg and her home in Washington, D.C. I was gone for weeks at a time and consequently really had not settled into my new surroundings. When I was home, it seemed that I was always busy preparing for my next trip. After my mother died, I was shattered and needed a reprieve from sadness and drama. I wanted to write, paint, and make new friends. I wanted to travel, begin to enjoy life once again and wake up from what felt like a bad dream. I certainly did not want to jump from the frying pan into the fire.

But Nan did come to live near us and in the end my personal issues were nothing at all when compared to the sorrow I have felt watching Nan mentally deteriorate. Accepting her fate has been a daunting journey. Frankly, there have been moments when I have been brought to my knees and almost shattered by the hopelessness of it all. Who is this woman who in a split second can become mean, aggressive, loud, and vulgar? Who is this woman whose language would make a sailor blush?

And most importantly, how could I ever learn to understand and accept the person she was becoming?

Initially I played the game of nonacceptance. I was a scout who was constantly on the lookout for proof that she was not declining. I looked for tiny remainders of her old personality. Any evidence, no matter how small, would make my heart leap. All she had to do was say a phrase in the old way, or give me her customary wink-of-the-eye, and I would emotionally drop everything and run back to her with my arms outstretched like a greedy child. But sadly I was always disappointed. Her familiar responses only proved to be an illusion, like a sleight of hand trick that lasted for an instant before vanishing into thin air. Her actions were nothing but reflexive responses that had seeped through tiny fissures in her new personality. So I would have to begin again, forced to face the fact that the diagnosis had been correct all along. What I had thought was a reawakening was nothing more than the final sputters of a flickering candle just before it dies.

If you have ever cared for someone you love who is suffering from a progressive illness, I am certain that you have found yourself trapped in this same cycle of false expectations and inevitable disappointments. My happiness was always short-lived and it was never long before reality crashed down on me, shattering my hope into a million tiny pieces at my feet. I have come to learn that this respite in Nan's erratic behavior was only the natural ebb and flow that occurs with gradual mental deterioration.

Looking back I can see that even though my intellect understood the reality of the situation, it took time for my heart to catch up with my head and accept what was occurring. My wishful thinking had conspired against me and dramatically altered how I interpreted Nan's actions and behaviors. I found what I wanted to find. But who can blame me? After all, when you don't want to face a painful truth, *wishes* and *hopes* cast powerful spells.

If today you find yourself caught in this same cycle, don't despair because there is a bright side to all of this crashing and burning. Unbeknownst to me, while I was experiencing the continuous cycle of hope and disappointment, I was slowly gaining ground, nudging my way through my fears and anxieties, inching my way toward accepting the truth. With each turn of the wheel I was chipping away at my unrealistic hope that Nan would be restored. It took time, longer than I would care to admit, but eventually I accepted her new reality. And this brought me an extraordinary peace, like a ceasefire that comes after a hard-fought battle.

Nan's official diagnosis of dementia forever changed the lives of everyone in our family. I remember sitting with my husband in a row of metal chairs along the hallway in a medical facility while she was being examined by a geriatric neurologist. It seemed to take an eternity. Finally the doctor emerged from the scan room and told my husband and me, "She has significant brain shrinkage indicating dementia or Alzheimer's disease. There is not much we can do at this point. There are medications, but their effectiveness is questionable. Her situation is progressive and will probably worsen over time."

Neither one of us was surprised. Our concerns had finally been verified. Then two questions immediately came to mind. First, how were we going to provide her with the care she was going to need in the future? And secondly, how were we going to help Nan understand the reality of her diagnosis? It was in these mind-numbing moments that I began my journey into the complicated world of dementia care. Its complexities were unimaginable and I knew its future was unpredictable. And I was afraid; afraid for Nan and afraid for us. The only thing I knew for certain was that Nan's cognitive skills were diminishing at an alarming rate and she needed help, now.

Watching Nan slip down through the stages of her dementia has been like witnessing two deaths simultaneously. I know this may sound emotionally counterintuitive. Either someone is here or they are not. But this is not the case when someone suffers from dementia. A schism occurs between the mind and the body.

For long after the mind fades and becomes just a trace of what it used to be, the body remains standing sentry like an abandoned house that has been weathered to a dusty pale gray. It is now a mere shell of what it used to be. The occupants that once lived there moved on long ago and all that remains are the ghosts of past inhabitants. The rooms that were once filled with the laughter and chatter of everyday life are now silent, except for the occasional creaking of an iron hinge as a shutter bangs against the peeled siding. Yes, the house is there for you to visit, but it now sits far back off the road, surrounded by gnarled hardwoods and waist-high weeds. If you squint hard enough you can still make out what it looked like in its finer days. If you listen closely you can hear the sound of children playing and experience the quiet peace of a summer's day after the noon meal. And this is all you have to sustain you for the many years it will take until this shell and its inhabitants are reunited for eternity.

I don't know when Nan began to separate from the world. I can't put my finger on the time when her disease finally overtook her mind, and I don't know if it even matters. But I do know that it seems to have happened in the blink of any eye, sometime when I wasn't looking. Dementia will trick you like that. It distracts you with its initial symptoms that send you scurrying about on endless missions to solve daily problems and search for cures. It sneaks up behind its victims and snatches them while you are busy making sure that they are taking their medicine correctly and eating a balanced diet.

Eventually Nan's decline became so evident that it could no longer be ignored. Her bad moments began to outweigh her good ones, forcing me to realize that nothing and no one could change the course of her disease. I felt helpless in the fight. My opponent had won. All I could do was brace myself and try to make every moment we spent together as positive and memorable as possible. Instinctively I knew that I was running out of time, so I strived to create memories that would sustain me through the dark days that I knew were fast approaching.

Not one of us gets through life unscathed. As a matter of fact most of us mark our lives by both our joys and our sorrows. If we are lucky the weights stack higher on the side of happiness. We all suffer setbacks, disappointments, and personal losses. I certainly have. Dear friends have died suddenly. Both my parents passed away after enduring long painful years battling cancer. I was unable to have the family I had always desired. And like so many baby boomers, I have been forced to say goodbye to the majority of my family members from the World War II generation.

Farewells are never easy for any of us to bear. Whether permanent or brief, some goodbyes are bittersweet, a mingling of sorrow with joy. I lived the first five years of my life in foster homes and even on that glorious day when I went to live with my new parents, I remember feeling both happy and sad. I was sad to leave all those I had come to love, but grateful to have found a family that I could call my own. Like most goodbyes, my first was an odd mixture of gratitude and sorrow.

This is much how I feel concerning Nan's dementia. I am thankful that she is still physically here, but I can't help but grieve her vanishing personality and the woman that she once was. Accepting the death of her identity has been a long and painful process. No matter how many loved ones we have lost, or how many goodbyes have been forced upon us, we must once again go through the grieving process, a process that has no shortcuts. We have to walk through the pain. We must keep trying over and over by placing one foot in front of the other until we reach a place of peace.

When someone you love dies you miss all the elements that make them unique—their quick wit and depth of spirit or their wicked sense of humor. You miss seeing their smile, holding their hand, or looking into their eyes. You miss every element that encompasses the totality of their person, both physically and emotionally. And for a long time, even after they are buried, your subconscious continues to search for them. Everywhere you go, there is a part of you that hopes that they will turn up and it was all just an awful practical joke, a great mistake.

I cannot count how many times after I lost my father that I thought I saw him on a street or in a crowd. A fierce flash of longing would overtake me until an unfamiliar gentleman would turn and show his face, leaving me bewildered and swallowing hard to push down the lump in my throat.

This is very similar to what it is like to be with a dementia patient every day. You see them sitting in a chair looking much the same as they always have and your heart leaps, thankful just to be able to spend time with them. And yet again that glimmer of hope pushes up from your heart. Maybe, just maybe, things aren't what they seem. But soon, before you know it, an odd remark or unnatural gesture pulls you backward and reminds you that they have indeed changed. This momentary hope only makes the reckoning all the harder and the path forward a steeper climb. It is like a wound that is never permitted to completely heal.

I wish I had a way to spare you the highs and lows of the acceptance process. I wish that I could catapult you past the pain and make you see the happiness that is possible even in the light of all that you are facing.

But I know that this is impossible. So instead, I will offer you the lessons that I have learned and hopefully they will make a difference.

Dealing with Nan's mental decline has been a balancing act of epic proportions. While grieving the loss of her personality, I have worked tirelessly to celebrate the continuation of her physical life. Over time I have learned to see those rare moments when her old personality peeks through, not as evidence of her restoral, but instead as the fuel I need to keep moving forward. Those moments motivated me to work even harder to keep the connection alive. They have become the joys that have helped me overcome my frustrations. By being honest about her prognosis and dissecting my feelings as a caregiver, I have been able to direct my energies in a positive direction. By accepting her situation, I have braced myself for what I know lies ahead. By deciding to drink in every minute of our long goodbye, I've created a new hope that our journey will continue for a long time to come.

In 1969 Elisabeth Kübler-Ross published her now famous book entitled *On Death and Dying* in which she details the five emotional stages of grief that are experienced when an individual is faced with impending death or other catastrophic life event.[1] She argues that bereavement is a universal experience shared by all of mankind and is not just applicable to death. In actuality, it is possible to experience grief as a result of a variety of life situations. Ms. Kübler-Ross also notes that these stages are not necessarily a complete list of all possible emotions that can be felt in the grieving process, nor do they have to appear in the order in which they are presented in her book. She also explains that the intensity of each stage will vary between individuals.

THE KÜBLER-ROSS FIVE STAGES OF GRIEF

Denial—In this stage we refuse to accept the reality of a given situation and instead utilize denial as a defense mechanism. Typically it is the reaction that carries us through the first wave of our pain.

Anger—Once we are no longer denying the reality of the catastrophic situation, the pain can often reemerge in the form of anger. The anger can be aimed at objects, strangers, family, or friends. Anger can even be directed toward the person who is ill or dying.

Bargaining—When we feel helpless and vulnerable we often resort to bargaining in order to try to regain a sense of control. We may try to make a deal with God or higher power, promising that we will make changes in our life if the situation is remedied.

Depression—There are two types of depression that are associated with the grieving process. The first is a reaction to the practicalities of the given situation. Will there be enough money to pay the bills? Will I be able to provide adequate care for the individual who is ill? The second type is more private and subtle. It surrounds the fear that comes from knowing that we soon may be separated from our loved one.

Acceptance—Acceptance occurs when we no longer feel anger and denial. Although not necessarily at peace, we have accepted the reality of our given situation. We realize that the truth cannot be altered and we begin to prepare ourselves for the inevitable.[2]

I first discovered Ms. Kübler-Ross's model when my father was facing a terminal illness in the late 1970s. After reading her book I was deeply moved, not only by the stories of the terminally ill patients that she studied, but also by how accurately she depicted the stages and feelings that I was facing. I was barely twenty years old and had never experienced a loss of this magnitude. It was as if she had looked inside my head and taken notes on my thoughts and emotions. The wisdom of her book has stayed with me ever since and has been the catalyst to understanding other significant losses and disappointments in my life, like learning to accept Nan's illness.

This model reminded me that my changing feelings were a natural part of the acceptance process. When I felt trapped, lonely, and selfish, I would examine my emotions in relation to the stages detailed by Ms. Kübler-Ross. Consequently, I gave myself permission to experience a myriad of negative and positive feelings as they arose. Her model served as my framework for healing and guaranteed me that, although I needn't push myself, it was imperative that I continue to work toward acceptance. I just needed to be patient and give myself time to mentally process the situation. If I did, my understanding would evolve naturally.

For me *anger* was the most difficult stage of my journey to acceptance. I know from spending time with other caregivers that this is often the case. Anger is a natural emotion and stumbling block when a loved one is diagnosed with a disease that causes progressive cognitive impairment. This also seems to be the stage in which many people become stuck, and I can understand why. For unless you have dealt with it personally, it is impossible to comprehend the devastating impact this kind of disease has on the daily life of everyone around the patient. You are never free of it. It is omnipresent. Even when you are engaging in other activities, it lurks in the corner, sneering at you, stealing your happiness and peace. You are forever waiting—waiting for a new problem to arise, waiting for a new symptom to develop, and waiting for the other shoe to drop.

My solution was to try to take the focus off myself and concentrate solely on what was best for Nan. I don't mean to sound saintly or self-righteous. On the contrary. I have had to struggle and fight hard against anger and frustration for many years. No, it is just that I have found that I feel better when I concentrate on what I can add to Nan's life, instead of what is being subtracted from mine.

Nan was still able to walk with the aid of a cane when she lived in her first memory unit. In those days I would receive no less than five calls a week notifying me that she had either hit someone with her cane or was using it to trip other patients as they passed by. This always happened at the most inconvenient time possible, but I would drop everything and dash over to the facility to try to appease the situation. I cannot tell you how many embarrassing conversations I have had with the family members of patients whom she had tried to harm. I would apologize for what she had done and guarantee them that I would do everything in my power to get her under control. But this was easier said than done. At one point, I even worried that she might be sued!

I can still hear myself pleading with her, "Please, never, under any circumstances touch anybody else." My demands were ineffective and fell on deaf ears. Either she felt that the other patient deserved it, or she had completely forgotten the incident by the time we sat down to discuss it. Her doctors tried to relax her through the use of drug therapy, but she became lethargic and wanted to sleep all day, which caused her to miss important meals. Finally the staff and I decided that it would be best if she spent as much time as possible in her room, away from other patients who seemed to trigger her hostility.

Luckily she never seriously hurt anyone; thank goodness the aids always stepped in before the situation had gone too far. However, the more I was forced to cope with the daily madness that swirled around her, the angrier and more frustrated I became. Honestly, I wanted my old life back. I found myself resorting to prayer in an attempt to remain even-keeled. I kept telling myself that Nan was not trying to drive me crazy, it just felt that way. I had to learn to stand back and look at things clearly. I mean, how could I hold a grudge against someone who has absolutely no idea what they are doing? But for a very long time my internal anger was difficult to quell. It took logic, time, and reasoning for me to win my fight against anger.

The road to accepting a diagnosis of dementia has as many paths as there are people facing this challenge. As you can imagine, over the many years that I have been caring for Nan, I have met and formed strong bonds with other family members in circumstances similar to mine. I have been able to observe firsthand how different people react to the same situation. I have witnessed the entire gambit of emotional reactions when family members are faced with this diagnosis. Some relatives accept the truth immediately and try to help in any way that they can, while others simply refuse to see the reality of the situation and argue with the patient and other family members. Others give up, turn their backs, and walk away.

I cannot speak to the complexities of acceptance without mentioning that there is someone else who is also going through this process. I am not the only one trying to come to grips with Nan's diagnosis. Nan is also transitioning through her own grieving process. In the beginning, when she was still able to think logically, she was fully aware of her deficiencies. She knew that something was terribly wrong with her mind. She knew that her thoughts were no longer clear and logical. On numerous occasions she told me that she thought that she was "going crazy" and wasn't "thinking straight." Sometimes when she said this, she would hastily grab my arm, as if this critical information had to be relayed quickly before her confusion returned. Her voice would croak in desperation and her eyes would dilate with fear. It was as if she was begging me to save her—from the world and from herself. These exchanges still haunt me to this day.

I'd like to think that as time passed, within the depths of her heart she eventually achieved some semblance of acceptance, and if not complete acceptance, at least a quiet peace regarding her situation.

Although I will never know for certain, there are times when I believe this may have occurred.

One afternoon while sitting in the courtyard of her first care facility, she was chatting and I was doing my best to keep pace with her nonsensical conversation. I was nodding my head and hopefully saying "Yes" and "I see" at the appropriate moments, when out-of-the-blue Nan turned to me, took my hand, looked me straight in the eye and with all the clarity in the world said, "I will be fine. Everything will be alright. It will be okay." I was stunned. Was she telling me what I thought she was? All I could do was sputter back, "Yes it will. I promise it will." And then she said the sweetest phrase in the English language. She said, "Thank you." And it was in that moment that I knew for sure that she and I would make it. We would figure it out. Somehow I would make things better. I would become her voice. I would fight for her. I had to. If she could accept this, so could I. Because if deep in the bottom of her battered soul she believed everything would be alright, how could I not believe it, too? How could I not set all my frustrations and worries free, like balloons sailing skyward? How could I not trust that, as Nan put it, "Everything would be alright?" And in the end, she was correct.

Knowing the reality of a situation does not prevent your heart from wishing that it wasn't so. When facing an emotional crisis, it often takes time for your heart to catch up with your intellect. You have to be patient with yourself. You may even have to fake it for a while and just go through the motions, getting the job done, while your emotions continue staggering in disbelief. But in the case of dementia, in order to effect positive change and improve both your situation and that of your loved one, you have to face the truth and let reason be your guide. I'm sorry but the doctors were correct all along. She will not get better. She will continue to decline, and there is nothing that I can do about it. It is out of my hands.

Now is the time to relax and have faith in the experts. Now is the time to have faith in yourself. Let yourself exhale. Prepare yourself for all the challenges that are heading your way. And when you have accepted the truth, you will have a new task. You will need to get busy and strive each day to find some semblance of joy in the midst of all this sorrow.

When I look back I can see just how far I have traveled. My progression has been natural and organic, like a quiet emancipator working hard to set me free until, at long last, the final piece of the puzzle slid neatly into place and I was able to fully accept and love this new Nan. I faced my truth head-on. I was the caregiver of a dementia patient who was never going to be whole again. And once I really knew this in my heart, I was able to begin to make a positive difference in Nan's life. I am proud to say that since this acceptance, there has been no stopping me.

I have no way of knowing how long Nan will be with me. One week? Three months? Five years? Only God knows. But I have come to hope that our final goodbye will be a long time coming, far in the distant future.

In my experience, the road to acceptance was not a linear trek. Instead it was filled with switchbacks and sharp turns and the occasional dead end. Over time it was reduced to a well-worn path filled with deep ruts and tear-filled furrows. But I continued to trudge those dusty roads again and again until at last, my pace quickened as the remembered peace of acceptance overtook me. And so I kept moving forward, ever-faster, leaving all the grief and fear in the hills that stretched far behind me, until I no longer felt the need to turn and look back one more time.

INSIGHTS

- Learning to accept that your loved one is suffering from dementia is a slow and individual process.
- Know that you are not alone in your sadness. Find comfort in the Kübler-Ross Stages of Grief.
- Understand that initially denying the diagnosis is a natural part of the acceptance process. Don't berate yourself if you keep searching for evidence that the diagnosis is incorrect.
- Don't go it alone. Seek support from family, friends, healthcare professionals, or an outside support group.
- Knowledge is power. Read all that you can about the progression of dementia so that you are prepared for what lies ahead.
- Interact with other caregivers in order to learn how they coped with the stages of their loved one's disease.

- Don't be hard on yourself. There is no straight road in your journey toward acceptance. You may transition through multiple stages several times before you are able to process your new reality.
- If your feel yourself stuck in any of the stages, don't be afraid to seek outside help so that you can move forward.
- Acceptance is easier if you stay focused on what remains of your loved one, instead of what has departed.
- Give yourself permission to grieve the loss of your loved one's personality.
- Remember that your loved one is going through their own version of the acceptance process.
- Realize that not everyone in your loved one's life will experience the stages of acceptance in the same way or at the same time. Be especially careful to respect where they are on their own personal journey.
- Keep your eye on the prize. Remain focused on the well-being of your loved one instead of counting and comparing each individual family member's contributions.
- Remember that it will take time for your heart to catch up with your head.
- Be patient with yourself and everyone in your loved one's life. Remember to act tenderly.

3

THE MOMENT BY MOMENT TECHNIQUE

All that is important is this one moment in movement. Make the moment important, vital, and worth living. Do not let it slip away unnoticed and unused.

—Agnes DeMille, quoting Martha Graham
Martha: The Life and Work of Martha Graham

We do not remember days. We remember moments.

—Cesare Pavese
The Business of Living: Diaries 1935–1950

Over the past ten years I have walked intimately with this disease called *dementia*. It has been my nemesis, my dilemma, and my unyielding opponent. It has been a source of incredible personal growth and a constant challenge. Not only have I witnessed Nan's advancing disease, but I have had the opportunity to observe countless other patients and their families fight the same fight. Some have won and some have not, but each person I have met along this arduous path has made me wiser and broadened my knowledge of the symptoms and effects of this devastating illness. I have found it impossible to visit Nan each day without becoming attached to other patients and learning from their family situations. Of course dementia's progression does not follow one set blueprint, but from my observation there are consistencies universal in all cases. It is from these constants that I derived my Moment by Moment approach to dementia caregiving. What began as small experimental activities grew into a much larger plan that eventually impacted every aspect of my time with Nan and hopefully made her life more meaningful.

This approach improves the life of both the patient and the caregiver. This is important because the act of caregiving involves a delicate balance between you and your loved one. The emotion of one participant absolutely impacts the well-being of the other. When Nan is content and at peace, I am calm and know I am doing my job. Likewise, if I am relaxed and happy during our visits, Nan tends to sense this and is more likely to be content and tranquil. Granted, there are times when nothing I do seems to calm the situation, but once I began implementing my approach it wasn't long before Nan's good days began to outnumber her bad days.

This technique is fluid and should be recalibrated as the patient's condition changes. You have to remember to remain flexible. Once you understand the fundamental principles, I am confident that there will be no stopping you. You will find yourself continually using these techniques in all aspects of your caregiving duties.

If I add up the columns in my caregiving ledger, joy and fulfillment far outweigh the stress and anxiety. This may sound hard to believe, but over time as my maturity and understanding grew, so did my expertise and tolerance. I learned that there are countless opportunities for Nan and me to share joy and create small triumphs. This is what I want for you. I want you to begin to experience the many wonderful surprises that can occur when caring for your loved one. This is your chance to tap into depths of courage and creativity that you never thought you possessed. This is your chance to discover talents that you would have sworn you never had.

Having found my way to this approach feels like nothing short of a miracle. Without it I truly don't know if Nan or I would be as happy as we are today. It has impacted every aspect of our relationship, from how I communicate with her, down to the priorities that I set each day. It has reoriented my compass. It has lifted our spirits and made joy possible.

My breakthrough began when I honestly assessed Nan's situation and my vision for her new restricted life. Of course my first concern was for her safety, but once this need was met I was determined that she find some semblance of happiness. At the time I wasn't sure exactly what that would look like, but I made it my goal to find out.

THE CAREGIVER

Let's begin with you. This may come as a surprise since up until this point you have spent the better part of each day tending to the needs of your loved one. I know all too well just how easy it is to become reactionary when daily challenges are thrust upon you. Of course, you will still need to solve problems as they arise, but I don't want that to be your sole purpose. Frankly, I am asking you to lighten up. I want to encourage you to spend less time problem solving and remember to include time for joy and fun. I can hear you now, "Fun? Are you crazy? There is nothing fun about caregiving." If this is how you truly feel, I encourage you to rethink your position and change your attitude.

Instead of viewing everything surrounding your loved one's care as a problem, I want you to spend time envisioning the vital and valuable person that they once were. I want you to look at your loved one from a different vantage point. I want to encourage you to see your purpose as a caregiver as more than someone who tends to physical needs. I want you to relax in order to release your creativity and sense of play. I want you to stop worrying about problems you cannot fix. Instead take hold of each small moment that you can control, and live it large! I want you to celebrate who your loved one once was. If you do, you will become more effective when meeting daily challenges and will find new ways to solve old problems. Why, you may even find enjoyment in the most mundane tasks. Take time to reexamine your caregiving approach and goals.

So much has been written about and discussed regarding the effect that attitude plays in our daily lives, that the concept itself has become a cliché. I can almost see your eyes roll into the back of your head at the mere mention of the word. But as is the case with most platitudes, they have become part of our cultural vernacular for one important reason. They are true. And attitude is no exception. In the world of caregiving, it is paramount—a factor that shapes the outcome and happiness of both you and the patient.

Many people operate under the false assumption that their attitude is a product of their situation, that they are a helpless victim to whatever problems life throws their way. They say, "If you had to deal with everything that I do, you'd be miserable too." Feeling this way turns us into victims. It makes us intolerant of new ideas and causes our actions to lose direction and purpose.

This emotional pitfall is particularly easy to fall into when you have to deal with a dementia patient every day. This thankless job is usually thrust upon you in a crisis situation, and is compounded by the fact that most of us have no experience dealing with someone who is mentally challenged. Consequently, it is all too easy to pity yourself and your predicament. Add in a healthy dose of family drama and a few financial worries, and your stress level rockets right off the chart.

Viktor Frankl was a holocaust survivor who had spent time in both the Theresienstadt ghetto and in the Auschwitz concentration camp. In his famous book, entitled *Man's Search for Meaning*, he writes the following: "Everything can be taken from a man but one thing: the last of the human freedoms—to choose one's attitude in any given set of circumstances, to choose one's own way."[1]

How you react is always your decision, yours alone. You must decide how you will behave. You must decide to make a difference. You must recognize that if you don't create joy and meaning in your loved one's life, no one else will. You must make it your goal.

If you had known me when I first began caring for Nan, you would have thought that my goal was to make myself as miserable as possible. I was the champion of self-pity. Most days I felt just plain sorry: sorry for me, sorry for Nan, sorry for my husband, sorry for how caregiving was taking over my life. After all, this was not how I had planned to spend my forties.

I continued like this for some time until I eventually reached the point when I was so sick and tired of being sick and tired, that I decided that enough was enough. If I were going to provide care anyway, why not have a positive attitude? In order to be happy again, I had to get tough with myself and lay down some ground rules.

Rule number one: I would not allow myself to think negative or deflating thoughts about myself, Nan, or my situation. When that old familiar destructive voice tried to sneak into my head, I banished it, threw it out, and kicked it to the curb. I refused to give it any power.

Rule number two: I tried to not let myself murmur or complain to anyone about any aspect of my caregiving experience. I found this to be the most difficult rule to follow, but in the end it proved to be the most profoundly helpful.

Rule number three: Each evening just before falling asleep, I would think of at least three positive moments or successes that had occurred during my time with Nan that day. Instead of lying in bed at night stewing about my sorry situation, I consciously decided to close my day on a positive note.

Needless to say, this was one tough assignment. I didn't just wake up one morning and stop the negative self-talk and complaining. Gratitude did not overtake me in an instant. No, it was a slow process—glacial in fact—but eventually I could feel myself modifying my feelings about being a caregiver. I did not realize it at the time, but I was redefining my role.

Once my attitude improved, my entire focus shifted. Instead of perpetually fixating on how the situation was impacting me, I tried to see myself as Nan's direct source for love, friendship, and support. Finally I began concentrating on what should have been my focus all along, to help Nan live the best life possible. From that point forward, I tried to approach my job as a caregiver with all the grace and honor that I could summon. I accepted that I had the power to better this situation. And today I am proud to say that caring for Nan has become my calling and my mission.

When you care for someone who has dementia, you are their eyes, ears, and voice in happiness and injustice. Caretaking is a huge job. But it is hard to be of use to anyone if you are constantly licking your wounds. Your reality has changed. Accept it, for both of your sakes. Stop focusing on yourself and unleash your creative energies onto the care of the patient. If you are able to do this, I promise that you will find rewards more plentiful than you ever could have imagined.

If you find yourself in the position I am, the odds are that you are somewhere in your middle years and have experienced both triumphs and setbacks during your life. You have probably labored in the outside world and experienced the richness of family life and the many joys of companionship. Cloak yourself in the successes of your life. Gather strength from the difficult times from which you triumphed.

The beauty of being middle-aged is that I have learned to ride the highs and lows of life with greater ease. I've learned when to pedal hard and when to coast. I believe in my power to positively affect the world around me. I believe in taking care of all the people who have loved me into being. I believe that if I strive to do every activity, no matter how small, with the greatest possible excellence, I will have lived up to my divine purpose. I no longer need accolades from the outside world to find the peace that comes from a job well done. I know now to recognize and be thankful for every little miracle.

If you have spent any time in the southeastern United States you have probably seen our live oak trees draped with ghostly Spanish moss. Languid as a slow, Southern drawl, this lichen dangles and gently sways in humidity so thick that you can almost cut it with a knife. In the spring when the moss is dressed in delicate antebellum flowers, you barely notice the strong oak that supports all this magnificent beauty. If you look closely, you will even see small resurrection ferns tucked in among the natural folds of the bark. I have always marveled at the live oak's ability to withstand these prolific freeloaders. But oddly, the tree is not harmed; instead it is the life force that enables all this beauty. When it rains the tree's nutrients wash down to feed the mossy canopy below, and so this kindred connection lives on. The oak stands as an unassuming support for the life that could not exist without it.

As the caregiver, you are also the source of all the possibilities that exist for your loved one. You are their shield against the ravages of an angry disease and a soft place for them to rest. When you stop and think about it, it is an honor and a duty so high that few people possess the courage or strength of spirit to take it on. To be needed at such an extraordinary level is both beautiful and frightening at the same time. Embrace all the sacred richness that this experience can bring into your life. Believe me it is a challenge that you will someday be glad you accepted.

THE PATIENT

As the moments of our lives stream by at what often feels like breakneck speed, it is easy to take them for granted, barely noticing them for all their richness. We squander them recklessly, spending millions each day on unimportant or inane activities. We certainly don't worship or revere them, and seldom do we adequately calculate their value and importance. Oh, there are occasions when we instinctively want to capture and restrain them, holding them close, and stopping time, like when a parent lay dying or a new baby enters the world. Like fireflies on a summer's night, we want to capture these moments and place them in a jar on our bedside table so they will be there when we dream, and comfort us during our darkest nights.

When I look out at what lays ahead in my life, moments seem to stretch for as far as the eye can see. Their numbers are like a multitude, blurring together and losing their individual importance. Caught in life's continuum, it is easy to take small moments for granted and let them slip by unnoticed and unappreciated. However, they define my place in the moving stream of life, the constant conveyor belt that continually nudges me forward.

But for an individual who is suffering from dementia, time looks very different. They no longer have the ability to peer over their shoulder and see the recent past, nor can they see the landscape of their future days. Their only real clarity lies in their distant past when they were young and their world was new. Is it any wonder that they are confused? It is as if they are time travelers, torn from the years of their youth and hurled into the present day. The details of their everyday life lack clarity, like small patchwork fields seen from the window of a low flying airplane.

In 1938, playwright Thornton Wilder's iconic American play *Our Town* opened on Broadway. It takes place in the small fictional town of Grover's Corner, New Hampshire, in 1901, and the audience is invited to share in the lives of two families who become joined by the marriage of their children, George and Emily. Nine years later, Emily dies in childbirth and is buried in the town cemetery beside many people whom she loved in life. Against the urging of the others in the cemetery, Emily decides to revisit her life one more time, choosing the morning of her twelfth birthday in the house where she grew up. But she can only observe the morning bustle as an onlooker and cannot be seen or heard. As her mother attends to her morning chores, Emily is overcome with emotion, crying, "Mama, I'm here! Oh! How young Mama looks!" But she receives no answer from these shadows from her past. Throughout Act 3, Emily continually tries unsuccessfully to get her family's attention, until finally she is resigned to her fate and asks to be returned to the cemetery to rest among the others who have departed.[2]

So often when Nan is speaking of her mother and father, I think of this play. I think of Emily's frustration as she tries to speak to her parents who are no more real than the images on a newsreel. Like Emily, Nan is reliving a time that is gone, seeking responses that are no longer possible. I know from experience that most dementia patients continually search for their ancient past, reliving events and longing for people who left this world long ago. And when they don't find who they are searching for, they often become frustrated, depressed, and at times desperate. If you don't believe me, just spend some time in a special medical unit for the memory impaired and you will hear constant requests for mothers, fathers, and long-deceased spouses. Many patients even believe that those around them are long-lost family members. For many years, each time I saw a patient named Agnes, she would call me Bonnie and thank me for traveling all the way from Mississippi to visit her. Their minds become caught in a continuous loop of ancient memories, inside a world to which they would like to return, a world filled with people whom they love, miss, and desperately want to see again.

So what remains of the present for the dementia patient? This I can tell you with confidence and assurance. Moments. Brief, lovely interludes of time. They can no longer exploit them on their own, but as their caregiver, you can elevate them to greatness. Moments are just waiting for you to grab hold and begin using them in a productive way. They are your tools, your way in, the key that unlocks the deepest part of who your loved one used to be, and can help you regenerate their sense of play, laughter, and dignity. You can more effectively gain their cooperation. By creating a series of short-lived, momentary joys, even if only for an instant, you can offer them a semblance of peace and contentment.

You may be thinking, "Instant? I have to do all this work and attitude adjustment, just to gain instants?" And to this my answer is, "Yes!" Don't underestimate the power of an instant. All you have to do is witness your loved one's delight when they are listening to a beautiful Bach Cantata or helping you pot an heirloom tomato plant on a warm spring afternoon, and you will understand my meaning. You will soon become a believer. These insignificant instants will become the stuff of your future memories. You will come to cherish—yes I said *cherish*—sharing these small moments of grace with your loved one. And I want you to think about this cold, hard fact: These moments are really all you have. I decided a long time ago, that if Nan and I can only connect for short snippets of time, that was just fine with me. I am willing to meet her on her terms and create any form of connection that she and I can make.

And there is another reason why instants matter. After spending so much time with Nan in all stages of her disease, I have noticed this interesting fact: It is impossible for me to predict or discern which activities she will remember and which she will forget. This was particularly true in the early days of her disease. I cannot begin to tell you how many times over the years that Nan has amazed me by remembering events that occurred days earlier, activities that I never could have dreamed she would remember. One thing is certain: I should never underestimate her abilities or waste any opportunity to lift her spirits. Every moment is worthy of an attempt to elevate her existence. I've decided that I will inundate her with happiness whenever it is possible, knowing that some joys will stick with her and some will fall away. I don't care if only 5 percent of the happiness we share gets through; I've decided this is enough—enough to keep me going.

THE METHOD

Ask any business person how they get the job done and they will tell you that it is through the development of an intricate plan. Maybe it is my corporate background, but I believe that any plan worth its salt begins with a clear *mission statement*. I know that when you read the term *mission statement* your mind immediately turns to the board room of a large corporation and not to objectives that relate to your personal life. I would like you to rethink this.

When faced with any unique personal challenge, especially one in which we have no previous experience, creating a mission statement forces us to focus on the endgame, and what we hope to achieve. It strips away our unrealistic dreams and emotions, enabling us to work toward a specific outcome. It becomes the gauge by which all our actions are measured. My mission statement is my litmus test, serving as a scale against which I evaluate all of my caretaking actions. It has empowered me and forced me to focus on Nan rather than myself. I may not be able to stop the progression of the disease, but I can get busy, roll up my sleeves, and do everything I can to make her life better.

My Mission Statement

I will do everything in my power to maintain Nan's health, safety, and dignity, while adding meaning to her life by creating small moments of joy and happiness when we are together.

I hope my statement will inspire you to move forward with your own. You're going to need stamina and stick–to–itiveness in order to remain focused. But believe me; it is worth it in the end.

It is time to pause and rethink your approach. Stop the perpetual problem solving and consider a new plan, a new way of spending time with your loved one. If you do, you will find that the days ahead will not only be calmer, but will also be filled with mutual happiness.

I want to encourage you to create activities that will stimulate and bring joy to your loved one. Don't worry about making impressions that will last into the future. Instead maximize each moment that you are together by urging them to pursue interests and activities that they enjoyed in the past. If necessary modify the process to suit their current physical and cognitive abilities. Utilize every available moment to connect their minds and hearts to who they used to be.

How is your loved one currently spending their time? Whether they live in a facility or at home with you, closely examine their daily schedule and make an honest assessment. It is so easy to sit an inactive individual in a soft chair in front of a television set and fool yourself into believing that they are being mentally stimulated. In nursing homes, residents are often gathered in large groups to watch television. This is often where they spend the bulk of their day, either sitting quietly or napping out of sheer boredom. Sitting in one place for hours on end with no other stimulation than a television set, is not a life that any of us would chose. So let's take this squandered and wasted time and use it to make a difference in our loved ones' lives.

Nan has been exceedingly lucky to have lived in wonderful care facilities throughout her illness. We have all heard and seen the horror stories in the news, highlighting nursing home abuse and facilities so foul that they are almost uninhabitable. This has not been the case for Nan. Granted, we researched each facility thoroughly, checking state health scores and stopping in at various times of the day in order to check on patient care. And even after she became a resident we continued to diligently monitor her daily progress and activities. Our motto became, "Inspect what you expect."

It is important to remember that no matter how wonderful a facility is, in the end it is an institution geared for the systematic care of large groups of people. Their primary concerns relate to the patients' physical maintenance and their immediate medical concerns. Once this rudimentary care has been provided, there is often little time or resources to devote to the emotional well-being and happiness of each patient. Patients with memory impairment are often overlooked. Most facilities make a valiant effort to plan activities that will add substance and value to the lives of its residents, but nine times out of ten, the events planned are aimed at residents with the highest cognitive skills and abilities. And honestly this makes sense. It is easier to plan activities directed to their high-functioning residents. Bingo, board games, current news-of-the-day highlights, and jigsaw puzzles provide a modicum of stimulation for the greatest number of residents. Unfortunately, unless they are offered individual help, these activities are exclusionary and cannot be enjoyed by residents suffering from moderate or acute dementia. Even in the earliest stages of the disease, sufferers typically lack the focus and concentration to sequentially follow the rules of a game without assistance. Other than the occasional music program, dementia patients are usually relegated to the sidelines, unable to participate in the majority of a facility's activities. Therefore, I believe that it is our responsibility, as caregivers, to pick up where the facility has left off. It is our job to create and adapt activities specifically tailored to our loved one's interests and current proficiencies.

Now let's closely examine your loved one's limitations. Ask yourself, "What are their current mental capabilities? What are their physical and emotional limitations?" If you don't pay close attention to these questions and design your activities accordingly, there is a high likelihood that you will both end up extremely frustrated. This could turn a potentially positive situation into one of anxiety and failure.

In other words, I had to know what Nan couldn't do in order to maximize all the wonderful opportunities for joy that were still available to her. By accepting the negatives of her situation, I was free to turn my attention to all the wonderful possibilities that remained within her reach. If I wanted to create life-affirming experiences for her, I had to be honest in my assessment and recognize the borders that surround her world. I had to set up my parameters. She was my blank canvas and I wanted to make certain that my broad splashes of happiness covered the entire surface, right up to its edges.

If you think about it, it makes perfect sense. No gardener worth their salt would just walk out their back door, dig a hole, and plop a flower in it. First, they would stake the boundaries of their garden. Then they would study and learn their specific climate zone and the soil conditions so that the most optimal plants could be selected. Likewise, no mathematician or physicist would attempt to prove a complicated hypothesis by attaching values to the possible variables without first understanding the laws of nature and the applicable mathematical absolutes.

My starting point for change began the day that I set realistic expectations for Nan based on a correct assessment of her abilities within the parameters of her new reality. Change began when I recalibrated my expectations to align with Nan's current capabilities. By lowering the bar, I was setting her up for success and offering her the opportunity to connect once again to the world around her.

In order to correctly assess the patient's situation, you must ask yourself some basic questions: Can they walk? Are they able to follow simple instructions? Do they still recognize songs and their lyrics? Are they still able to use their hands to produce artwork? Can they still read, and if so are they able to interpret the words on a page? How verbal are they? Can they successfully express themselves? Do they remember their family members by name or when looking at old photographs? Does anything make them cry? Are they able to ride in a car? Do they need assistance in the bathroom? Are they able to feed themselves in a restaurant? Do they have uncontrollable outbursts when in a small group or out in a public setting? Can they begin activities on their own, or do they need someone to help them work through the process? What time of day are they most cooperative?

Keep in mind that the answers to these questions change constantly, sometimes from one week to the next. This is where flexibility comes into play. To be successful you must continually calibrate your activities to coincide with their ever-changing skill level. Nan and I used to be able to go for walks outdoors and look at the trees. But now, since she is relegated to a Geri-Chair, it has become necessary to take short strolls on the sidewalks outside her nursing home. Likewise, we used to play

CDs and sing folk songs and hymns together. Sometimes now the music will make her nervous and not offer her the pleasure that it once did.

When these setbacks occur, don't let them frustrate you, because oddly enough these situations always seem to take care of themselves. As Nan loses her ability to participate in an activity that once brought her joy, her enthusiasm seems to naturally move onto something else. For example, when Nan lost her ability to effectively communicate verbally through speech, her love for singing increased. For a short time she sang the answers to any questions that she was asked. I have only run into trouble when I have tried to push her to go beyond her current skills and dexterity.

Understanding and accepting the patient's limitations is the framework for the Moment by Moment technique. Once you understand this, you will feel as if you have been clued in on the secret rules of the game. And now the fun begins; you can let your creative juices flow.

There are as many possible activities as there are people who create them and people who enjoy them. To be successful you will need to do some brainstorming and reflect on your memories of your loved one. Begin by looking at old photos or ask other family members what they remember your loved one enjoying. Be a detective and look for the happiest times in their past. How did they like to spend their free time? If you want to connect with them on a deep level, you will have to personalize your approach by focusing on things that naturally delight and enthrall them.

At the end of this chapter, I have provided a list of questions that will help you begin your investigation. Of course, they are not inclusive but are simply tools that will help you begin to uncover the unique interests of your loved one.

Remember to think outside the box. If they love Greek food, have Greek food night. If they loved to entertain, share the evening with their friends at home or in the facility. If they loved spending time in London, prepare an English Tea for them one afternoon, complete with china cups, scones, and cucumber sandwiches. Again, the possibilities are endless. Try to remember the times when you saw your loved one the happiest. If they used to belong to a bowling league, consider purchasing a *Wii* bowling game that they could play in their room. I know for a fact that this can even be played from a wheelchair. Your goal is to reconnect them to who they used to be. Your goal is to bring a smile to their face, join in the fun, and love them not only for who they were, but also for who they have become. Your goal is to connect them to the world by maximizing small moments in time.

Yes, we both know that they will forget many of the activities that you plan. But who are we to say if the effect of joy is lasting? Who are we to say what fills a person's soul and offers them solace? And I ask you, what is our alternative? Sitting next to them watching television when we visit? I think not.

The beauty of this technique is that it can be applied to many aspects of your loved one's life. The Moment by Moment technique can be utilized to gain cooperation during simple everyday tasks. It works because you are breaking down and dissecting life into small pieces and doable steps that your loved one can better understand. I like to think that I am creating microsteps to joy and happiness.

I try every day to see the world through Nan's eyes. I try not to make judgments or cast any prejudices. I've had to push my vantage point into the back of my mind, and bring Nan's view forward.

In the chapters ahead, I will explain ways to connect the dementia patient to the most vital aspects of being human, those transcendent elements that touch us all: nature, spirit, dignity, and humor. For you see, even though your loved one has changed in many respects, deep inside they are just like you and me and are seeking love and peace. By striving to create small moments of happiness for them, you will find yourself releasing you own worries and fears, as if you are sending a calming prayer of joy out into the world.

When faced with the overwhelming pressures of caregiving, it is easy to lose your way and wander for a time in despair. When you are caught in the tedium of daily chores, it is easy to lose sight of your own power to create change. Viewing your situation through a lens of tasks and problems distorts and chokes out gratitude and hides all the possible beauty that remains available in your situation.

If you gaze at a sunset and only watch the sun, you will miss all the colors encircling the sky. Look around.

If you focus on just one flower, you will miss the splendor of the garden humming with drunken bees. Stand back.

If you only stare at the leaves piled on the ground, you will miss the barren beauty of silhouetted trees against the evening sky. Look up.

Don't miss this opportunity to create small joys for someone you love. Don't forget to set aside your chores and create wonderful memories that you can call upon in the future. Share happiness with someone you love before it is too late. Hurry up. The time is now.

INSIGHTS

- Individuals suffering from dementia still have the ability to experience joy and happiness.
- See your loved one's world in terms of small individual moments. Learn to take these moments and create delights for them and precious memories for yourself. Don't underestimate the power of an instant.
- Make it your goal to infuse your loved one's life with joy and meaning.
- Love them for who they are today. Join them in their world and don't try to drag them back into yours.
- Create your own personal caregiving mission statement.
- Investigate and find creative ways to celebrate your loved one's life and achievements.
- Remember that your attitude and outward emotions directly impact your loved one's behavior and happiness.
- Try to envision the world through the eyes of your loved one.
- Take time out of your caregiving chores in order to share pleasant activities with your loved one.
- Your attitude is not an inevitable product of your situation, but instead it is yours to create and control.
- Don't waste time complaining to others or thinking negative thoughts about your caregiving situation.
- Come from a place of gratitude. Remember to be thankful for all the miracles that you can still share with your loved one.
- Find strength from your past successes and achievements.
- Realize that we cannot predict what activities and experiences your loved one will hold in their memories. So do not waste any opportunity to lift their spirits.

- In order to create meaningful activities, analyze and understand your loved one's physical and cognitive limitations so that you can set them up for success.
- Turn off the television set and make your loved one's actual world interesting and engaging.
- Remain flexible and eager to adapt to your loved one's ever-changing skills as they progress through their disease.
- The Moment by Moment technique can be effectively utilized to gain your loved one's cooperation during simple everyday tasks.

THE MOMENT BY MOMENT TECHNIQUE

Questions to consider when developing joy-filled activities for the dementia patient include the following:

- Where was the patient born?
- What year was the patient born?
- What was the patient's occupation?
- How long were they married? Is their spouse still alive?
- Did they go to college? If so, what was their primary field of study?
- Did they serve in the military? If so, did they serve in wartime or receive any honors?
- Was religion an important part of their life?
- What community activities did they participate in?
- Did they enjoy music? If so, what kind?
- Did they paint, draw, or sculpt? Did they participate in an artistic hobby?
- Did they sew, crochet, or do needlework?
- Did they enjoy the outdoors?
- Did they like to hunt and fish? If so, where and for what game?
- Where have they traveled to in the world? What was their favorite country? Why?
- Did they enjoy dancing? If so, what kind?
- Who is their favorite author or poet?
- What subjects did they study throughout their life and never seemed to lose interest in? History? Art? Science? Astronomy?

- What is their knowledge of technology?
- Do they have an iPod or iPad?
- What was the best day of their life, and why?
- Did they like to sing? If so, what kind of music? Opera? Country Western? Folk songs? Hymns?
- What kind of volunteer work have they done in the past?
- What is their favorite holiday?
- What is their favorite season?
- What is their favorite flower?
- Do they have a favorite book they would like to revisit?
- Do they enjoy playing games? If so, which ones?
- Did they ever plant a garden? If so, what were their favorite plants to grow?
- Who is their favorite artist?
- What is their favorite movie?
- What were the happiest moments from their childhood?
- Did they play an instrument? If so, what instrument did they play?
- What is their favorite television show?
- Were they a supporter of a particular political party?
- Did they play sports? If so, which sport?
- Do they have a favorite sports team? If so, which one?
- Did they enjoy current events?
- Did they read a daily newspaper?
- What is their favorite magazine?
- What was the style and ambiance in their home?
- What is their favorite restaurant?
- Did they like to cook?
- What are their favorite foods?
- Do they have a favorite quote or Bible verse?
- Of all their personal possessions, which ones do they value most?
- Did they like to write letters?
- Did they have a pet?
- What movies or comedians make them laugh out loud?
- Did they have a favorite radio station? If so, which one? NPR? Oldies rock? Classical?

4

THE JOY CONTINUUM

There are only two ways to live your life. One is as though nothing is
a miracle. The other is as though everything is a miracle.

—Albert Einstein

Try as I might, I am not getting much work done at my desk this
afternoon. My mind is wandering. Looking out my window, instead of
my back garden I see my childhood home and the clear stream that ran
behind the house, and once again I feel the mud oozing between my
bare toes. So instead of working, I've been busy climbing trees and
eating chokecherries from a small pail filled with hose water. Indolence
has overtaken me, like a cat in need of a good long stretch.

Even through the window pane, I am distracted by the sounds outdoors—the maracas of cicadas, the sad call of mourning doves, and
Carolina wrens requesting a *tea-kettle-please*.

Despite the oppressive heat, the garden is bustling with activity this
afternoon. Striped bees are drunk from nectar, psychedelic butterflies
are vibrating against the green of the boxwood hedge, and swallowtails
are sailing overhead on summer's wavy, heat currents.

And Nan is here, too. Atop a pink china plate at the corner of my
desk, sits a gigantic blue mason jar that I found buried deep in the back
of her old hay barn. No longer canned with *Kentucky Wonder* beans
from her garden, it now holds beauties from mine: hydrangeas as big as
cats' heads, purple salvia blossoms still mourned by hungry bees, and
roses so tired that they must rest their heads on the lip of the jar, lest
they swoon. Even if it had come straight from a queen's private coffer,

no vase could be more treasured. I feel Nan near. Pieces of her life have trickled down to me, and she is everywhere.

Once again joy has snuck up on me, unplanned and gradual, like a breeze, a zephyr, warm and inviting. I wish that this feeling would last forever. But I know that it will leave soon enough, on the same wind that it blew in on, traveling in a two-seater biplane, wearing a skull cap and goggles, writing in the sky in white puffy letters, "Don't worry. I will return." But for now I will bask in this joy and pretend that it will never leave. I will be indifferent to winter's fast approach and ground soon frozen hard beneath purple moon shadows.

Wouldn't it be wonderful if we could live in a constant state of joy, when all the possibilities of the universe seem to lie at our feet? But we know that this is not possible. Joy is transient, never constant. The harder we try to capture it, the more likely it is to hide and evade our pleas for it to materialize. Joy is a sensation that cannot be forced, but instead it seems to appear when we least expect it, like an unexpected guest appearing at our front door bearing large suitcases filled with gifts from far-off lands. Joy is shy and rarely comes to call during times of great splendor and occasion. No, it likes quiet moments and tender scenes, far beyond the shouts and murmurs of this noisy world.

To worry is to be human. Throughout the course of our daily lives, we all worry. Some concerns are worthy of our attention, and some are not. Many anxieties are universal and touch each of our lives. Will I find a good job? Will I find a good mate? Will my children grow up to be healthy and happy? Sometimes these questions act as the fuel that propels us forward in pursuit of our life goals. However, if taken too far, worry can become destructive and overshadow all the wonderful possibilities that are present in our lives. Fear takes over when we are trying to solve the unsolvable or change the unchangeable. Once in place, it feeds on our darkest anxieties and shows its face in all we do.

Worry seems to go hand in hand with the enormous challenge of caring for a dementia patient. When we find ourselves accountable for the physical and emotional well-being of a helpless individual, our world is often fraught with anxiety and mind-numbing concerns. Each day in our battle with the disease, we are forced to perform a triage of sorts, constantly assessing and prioritizing the patient's current medical situation. If the proper care is not administered, they may become injured. At times our decisions are a matter of life or death. I don't know anyone in this situation who has not worried late into the night—eyes wide open, staring at a dark ceiling hoping that they are doing all they can to protect their loved one. We constantly audit every action and decision that we make. If we are not careful, soon we have stacked worry upon worry until we have built a ladder leading nowhere.

As caregivers, our lives are filled with countless issues that we cannot influence. We worry about the future of both the patient and ourselves. We worry about whether we have the stamina to continue on this treadmill called caregiving. We worry about what will happen when our loved one's financial resources run dry. We worry that the patient is losing too much weight. We worry that they may fall. We worry about how low their mental capabilities will plummet. Sometimes, I even find myself answering one worry with a new and even bigger worry. (For example, when I was concerned that Nan was losing too much weight, I began worrying about whether her meals were healthy and she was getting enough nutrition.) Worry upon worry, the list never ends. How could any semblance of joy creep into our lives when our minds are tied in knots of fear?

Guilt is another joy-stealer for the caregiver. It pops its head up everywhere. We have guilt that we are not doing enough, guilt that we can't change things, guilt that we are angry to be placed in this impossible situation, guilt for all the times we feel as if we need a break and guilt for those tiny moments when we secretly want to run away from home. To all of this, I say "STOP!"

In order to find any level of fulfillment and peace in this challenging situation you must do everything in your power to cast off your feelings of blame and fear. Guilt is not a mantle that any caregiver should wear. Just the fact that you have stepped up to the challenge makes you a hero, for heaven's sake. Just to have agreed to care so deeply for another individual, knowing full well how the story will end, takes great depth of courage and immense amounts of fortitude.

I want to awaken you to the idea that there is an alternative to this unhealthy anxiety. I want you to know that your daily life can look and feel very different from how it does today. Finding joy within the daily strains of the caregiving relationship, although difficult, is possible if you stay alert and direct your attention onto all that your loved one and you have accomplished. I know this works because I have done it. I had to learn to see each achievement, no matter how small, for what it really was—an incredible event.

Accept the principle that joy is possible in any situation, no matter how trying. Look around for joy. Hunt for it. Realize that joy travels to us via strangers, caregivers, patients, soft summer breezes, and sometimes even through special moments of our own creation.

I am not trying to make light of the effort that is required to make these changes. I know how difficult it is to look at dementia from the vantage point of joy. I am not suggesting that it is possible to dance your way through the caregiving experience bleary eyed and filled with bliss. On the contrary. It takes hard work and practice. However, I know from experience that inveterate worrying prevents us from seeing all the possibilities for joy in any situation, especially when fighting an opponent as colossal as dementia.

Caregiving is not for sissies. According to a 2010 study conducted at Catholic University in Leuven, Belgium, depression occurs in one in three caregivers and occurs more frequently in those who care for patients with dementia than those who care for individuals with other chronic illnesses.[1] Other studies have predicted that the rate of depression for caregivers is as high as 59 percent. I find these statistics a sobering motivation that urges me to continue searching for ways to cultivate happiness for both Nan and myself. Had I not altered my approach to caregiving, I am certain that I would have become yet another unhappy statistic. Changing directions saved my sanity, and was the seed from which I developed my Moment by Moment technique.

Remember that caregiving is a reciprocal relationship that cannot be effective unless the needs of both participants are considered of equal value. It is impossible to try to create joy for another individual when you are miserable yourself. I admit that in the case of dementia caregiving, joy can be a tricky emotion to find and almost impossible to maintain. But if you are observant and remain positive, it will burst upon you in the most unexpected moments, like a sudden rush of unscheduled hope.

Finding joy is not predicated on banishing all your feelings of fear and anxiety. I don't think that would even be possible. I am merely suggesting that you eliminate the worries that don't serve you well. Think small. Focus on what needs to be done today, during this hour, and not what lies ahead a year from now. For instance, my concern over

Nan's diet is valid since it is an issue that impacts her daily life and one that I am able to control right now. However, my worry as to how far she will mentally decline is an issue that I can clearly do nothing about. Focusing on it will only increase my stress level and distract me from what I need to accomplish today.

I have found that by staying attentive to what I am able to impact in the short term, I maximize Nan's chances for good health and well-being in the future. If I work hard to ensure that Nan receives the best possible medical care for this one day, I safeguard her future and have done my job well. Each morning I make the conscious decision to concentrate on that day, and let all my worries regarding tomorrow take care of themselves. In the end, I know that this is all I can do.

This approach lifts me up and allows me to lay down the burdens that have weighed so long on my shoulders. It makes my job manageable, and graces me with the control I need to actually make a difference in Nan's life. Energy that I had previously spent on nonproductive worries can now be spent focusing on the positive aspects of our relationship. Creating optimistic activities is difficult on our best day, but almost impossible when we carry the weight of the world strapped to our shoulders.

Understanding that joy is not a derivative of any specific circumstance unleashes the possibility that it can occur in some of our darkest moments. When it graces us with its presence, we have no concern about tomorrow, or even the next minute. We are living in the wonder of one particular fragment of time and seeing it in all its perfection. Even in the depths of despair it can show its face, offering hope and peace for one small period of time.

What a beautiful coincidence. If joy spontaneously shows its face for small sacred moments and our loved ones see the world in small sacred moments, what could be more perfect? A fantastic opportunity for happiness has been laid at our feet.

A few years ago, searching for a slideshow of our trip to Charleston, I was looking through a stack of DVDs that I had downloaded from our video camera. At the very bottom of the pile was one marked *Nan*. Was it from one of her birthdays? When was this taken? I slid it into the machine and pressed the *play* button. I couldn't believe my eyes, or rather, I couldn't believe my ears.

There was Nan sitting in a wheelchair in our back garden, and she was talking. Not the gibberish that she speaks today, but honest to goodness talking. She and my husband were discussing the flowers and laughing. She kept interrupting him in order to say how much she loved being outdoors in the sunshine. I was fascinated, mesmerized. I had forgotten all about that afternoon. I couldn't take my eyes off the screen. Wait, was that a joke she just told, a bit of wit? Did she just call us by name and laugh out loud? I was witnessing joy, Nan's joy. She was so happy and grateful to be spending the afternoon outdoors that her happiness was almost palpable. Nothing mattered to her but that one afternoon—the sunshine and spending time with her son. For those few hours, she was a woman with no problems.

Unfortunately, it was painfully obvious that my husband and I were not active participants in all this happiness. I could tell that we were seeing these events through a veil of worry and anxiety. I could see it on my husband's face. He was probably thinking about getting her home in time for dinner, while I know that I was probably busy praying that she wouldn't have to use the ladies room anytime soon. We were missing it. We weren't appreciating the glorious beauty of being able to spend an afternoon talking with Nan. Yes, I was thankful that we had made her afternoon pleasurable, but I was sad that we had chosen not to join in. We had missed out on all that joy.

I wanted to jump inside the picture and take both of us by the shoulders and shake us—shake us hard, shake us into mindfulness. I wanted the man sitting in the Adirondack chair and the woman behind the camera to stop worrying and appreciate the miracle that was before them. I wanted to shout, "Don't worry. It will be alright. Look at her. Talk to her. Ask her to tell you about the best day of her life. Tell her how much you love her. Thank her for every little thing that you can think of. Be grateful for this glorious moment, because things in the future will get much worse. Appreciate what you have right now."

When the disc ended I sat for some time thinking of how much Nan had changed. When I asked myself if I was still behaving this way, I decided that yes, I probably was. No parable or Aesop's fable could make it any clearer. It was like a bucket of cold water had been dumped on my consciousness. That afternoon in our backyard, I had been thinking only of myself and my role during her visit. I can't believe that I had wasted precious time worrying about the ladies room! I wasn't listening to Nan and I certainly wasn't watching her. Nan was presenting us with a precious gift, the knowledge that we had made her day a bit brighter, and we had been too self-absorbed to notice. Joy had been present and placed before me on a silver platter and I had missed it. I hadn't paid any attention.

How many other times had I let joy float by unnoticed? And what joy was I missing now, right now, this very day?

This instance taught me to stay alert and watch the landscape, because like a timid fawn that can quickly dart back into the shade of the forest, joy is easily spooked. I need to remember that joy is best shared. I need to remember to relax and sprinkle a bit of it on myself from time to time. I need to remember that each day that Nan is with me is a blessing and that I should seek my prize. After all, Nan's moments of joy are my reward and the fruit of my hard labor. Why would I leave one precious morsel of it rotting on the ground?

One question that I am frequently asked by well-meaning friends is, "If Nan is in a facility, why do you go and visit her so often? After all, it is not as if she even knows that you are there. Does it really make any difference whether or not you visit her?" I tell this story as my reply:

One afternoon five years ago Nan presented me with a gift of incalculable value. After sitting together for a few hours in the community room of her assisted living facility, I told her that I would have to be going home soon since it was almost time for dinner. As an afterthought, I explained that I had bought her two new blouses and that I had hung them in her closet. As I was turning to leave, she called after me with all the clarity of bygone days, "Everything I have that is beautiful is because of you." This random comment has stayed with me ever since and has lifted me up when I have felt tired and defeated. Unknowingly, Nan had passed on her joy to me and I was grateful. She once again had taught me a valuable lesson—to always leave the door wide open so that joy can find its way home.

According to a study conducted by Esther Oh, MD, of Johns Hopkins Memory and Alzheimer's Treatment Center, while depression in older adults is estimated to range from 7–36 percent, this number increases to 15–50 percent for individuals suffering from dementia.[2] She cites that depression in dementia patients often goes unnoticed because they are less likely to have trouble sleeping and often lack the ability to express their feelings of worthlessness or guilt. However, she states that they are more likely to become agitated, experience fatigue, and suffer from delusions and hallucinations.[3]

This was certainly the case for Nan. Since she had been diagnosed with depression prior to the onset of dementia, we watched closely for any evidence that her condition was worsening. Over time she began crying regularly and experiencing frequent hallucinations. It soon became necessary to modify her medications in order to effectively treat her worsening condition. In conjunction with her new drug regime, I implemented my Moment by Moment behavioral approach and began creating activities to boost her overall happiness. In Nan's case, these two therapies worked in unison to improve her mood and frame of mind.

It was about this time that I created a "Happy List" that Nan and I read during my visits. It consists of small universal pleasures that each of us have experienced sometime in our lives. What began as a brief assignment soon encompassed the better part of a large spiral notebook. I listed things in it that would call to mind happy thoughts and memories.

Here are some examples from my list: ice cream cones, new shoes, a baby's laugh, puppies, laying in a hammock on a summer's day, walking in the woods, an unexpected letter from an old friend, listening to a favorite song, grandchildren, a fresh bed dressed in cool crisp linens, a clothesline hung with lace curtains flapping in the breeze, flying kites, the poems of Robert Frost, a wedding invitation, a parade, fireworks, watermelon on a hot day, warm tomatoes eaten straight off the vine, dogwoods in bloom, the cry of the whip-o-will, rainbows, daisy chains, horses in a field, the sound of an orchestra tuning their instruments before a performance, the smell of fresh mown grass, birthday parties, Christmas morning, star gazing, the sound of rain falling on a tin roof, spring's first hyacinth, porch lights at night, going barefoot, making a wish as you drop a penny in a wishing well, picnics, the beautiful blue of a robin's egg, the face of someone you love. Our list went on and on.

We always took time to read from our notebook whenever we were together. Sometimes we would linger over one particular item and give it extra thought or share specific memories. As I read, neither of us could help but smile. This is just one example of how a small, simple activity can create a shared moment of pleasure. Over time it became a kind of gratitude journal. Every time I spotted some small miracle in my daily life, I would think, "I'll have to put that on the Happy List." It wasn't long before I had compiled hundreds of reasons to be grateful. To this day, when I see a perfect sunset or a turtle on the lawn, I think of Nan and our list.

Today, even though Nan is well into the later stages of dementia, we still play a variation of this game. I no longer read from our list, because too many thoughts and ideas would only confuse her. But when we are together, I find myself inventorying all the blessings that are surrounding her at that moment. If it is sunny, I comment on the beautiful weather. If it is raining, I am thankful that the lawn and the garden are being watered. I point out how lucky we are to have lunch served to us, and how lucky we are not to have to do the dishes. I explain that she is safe and that we are all well and happy. I comment on how cozy we are, and most importantly, how lucky we are that the Dear Lord has blessed us with yet another beautiful day. She no longer is able to offer appropriate verbal responses, but she smiles and nods in rapt appreciation.

What I am telling you is to never give up. Never underestimate the power of small joy-filled connections. Know that even though you are facing one of the hardest episodes of your life, deep down, beneath all the loneliness and fear, lay tiny sprigs of joy, much like snow drops that emerge from beneath a winter's snow. But remember, joy is demure and can easily be overlooked.

Always remember to set a place for joy at the table of your life, for you never know when he might decide to return. For just when you least expect it and you are certain he will never come again, you will hear the sputtering of that ancient biplane far off in the distance. Excitedly you will drop everything and run outside through the banging screen door, shielding your eyes from the setting sun, searching the skies for that old familiar friend. And suddenly you will see him emerging from behind the clouds, his goggles gleaming in the sun, his white scarf flapping behind him in the wind, and he is smiling down on you, giving you the thumbs-up, as he circles your field looking for a place to land.

INSIGHTS

- Joy is possible in any situation, even within the daily strains of your caregiving responsibilities.
- Don't give in to the joy-stealers. Work hard to push your fear and worry to the side so that there is room in your life for the joy that is occurring right now, today.
- Hunt for joy in your caregiving experiences—through strangers, caregivers, patients, and the beauty of the world around you. Look for it.
- Learn to enjoy your loved one right where they are today. Be thankful for any happiness that you are able to share.
- Don't be afraid to seek help if you have uncontrollable feelings of depression.
- Take the time to create avenues of joy for your loved one by exposing them to art, music, and nature.
- Pay attention. If your loved one thanks you or tells you they love you, make it a point to store it in your heart. For the day may come when they cannot convey these loving emotions.
- Be on the lookout for signs of depression in your loved one. If you suspect that they are depressed, speak to their doctor immediately.
- Create your own Happy List of life's simple pleasures and read them aloud to your loved one.
- Always remember to stay true to your mission statement. Make joy the focus of all your visits.

5

A POSITIVE APPROACH

Few things in the world are more powerful than a positive push—a smile. A world of optimism and hope.

—Richard M. DeVos

I awoke early this morning, long before the first blush of dawn, and lay in my bed listening to the last whispers of night. I was thinking of how far Nan and I have traveled and the countless challenges that we have faced together. Some have been small, while others have been monumental. Together in our tiny boat called *Hope* we have navigated the great rushing river of dementia. While traversing jagged rocks and currents so powerful that I often felt rudderless, I held firm to my belief that eventually we would come to rest among the calm reeds on the far bank. And this is where we are this morning, moored in a quiet spot where the waters are still and giant grasses quell the torrents of my worry and fear. Optimism and courage dwell along these shores, inspiring the wisdom and peace necessary to continue on our journey. And here we sit, waiting to be pushed on by the soft winds of time, hoping that the whirling gales of unhappiness lay far behind us.

The peace that I feel this morning is not that of a victorious conqueror. By now, I know all too well that dementia is a shifty opponent. I know that I cannot control every aspect of Nan's life and that I am only experiencing a temporary lull in her symptoms. I recognize that new problems will soon arise, that her disease might stabilize or it might worsen, and that someday critical physical ailments will overtake her body. I even understand that at some point in the future she may become blank and unable to communicate with anyone. And yet for now at least, I am at peace.

There is an old saying that I have learned to live by. "Just control the controllables." I realize that I cannot change the inevitability of Nan's situation. Despite my innumerable efforts, I always return to my mission statement and the realization that I can only control small moments within the confines of her ever-shrinking world. No heroic act or incredible epiphany will propel Nan back in time to who she once was. At the end of the day, as with most life experiences, all I can control is my attitude.

I am the filter through which Nan sees the world. My moods and behaviors influence how she interprets everything in her life. If I strive to be kind, she will know that she is loved. If I appear strong and in control, she will know she is safe. If I choose to be positive, I will show her there is hope.

Admittedly, at first it was difficult to maintain a positive outlook. I worked hard to remain optimistic, but sometimes her unstable behavior was too much to bear and a kind of helpless depression would overtake me. Those were hard days that brimmed with anger and resentment, and all I could do was walk away and begin again later.

No matter how hard you try, no positive approach leads you in a straight line. Instead, it ebbs and flows as the circumstances of dementia change. During these difficult times, you must take a breath and value all that you have achieved up until this point. Don't compare your loved one's behaviors against how they behaved yesterday, or how you hope that they will conduct themselves tomorrow. Instead, try to remain calm and give yourself credit for all the positive changes that you have been able to facilitate. Remember, this situation is never solved and its future will always remain uncertain.

Typically when I am feeling especially negative, it is because I have been focusing on the symptoms of the disease, rather than working to counterbalance its hold on Nan. It occurs when I am once again interpreting her actions in the context of who she used to be. It occurs when I forget that nothing in this life is permanent and that we don't have to understand everything that is happening around us in order to find happiness

The reality is that there will be times when you feel sad and hopeless. There will be days when you want to walk away. This is when you have to mentally grab hold of yourself and deliberately change the thoughts that are running through your mind. Sometimes I redirect my thoughts by saying affirming statements out loud. Sometimes a good night's sleep does the trick. Sometimes I go for a walk to clear my mind, go to dinner with a friend, or engage in an activity that I enjoy. I give myself permission to rest physically and emotionally. I remind myself that there is an entire universe outside the world of dementia.

Over time if you *decide* to remain positive it will become a habit. Yes, I said *decide*. For even with a diagnosis as horrific as dementia there are truths worth celebrating. And once I decided to open my eyes to all that remains possible, I began to see a multitude of tiny miracles swirling around Nan. I have witnessed more spontaneous demonstrations of kindness, understanding, and spirit-filled behavior than I can count. I didn't notice them at first. I had to learn to pay attention in order to see them. And to think that they were there all along, hiding behind the distractions of my daily life, just waiting to be detected and appreciated. Even in the advanced stages of her disease, there is so much about Nan's life to celebrate.

Nan still has the capacity to experience love and happiness.
Nan can still laugh and enjoy being with her family.
I still have time left to be with Nan.
Nan's new reality, although limited, still holds many wonders.
I have an opportunity to return the love that Nan has given me.
I know that Nan strives hard each day to remain engaged with the world around her.
Nan is loved by everyone she encounters.
By helping Nan I have become a better person.
Nan still has the capacity to enjoy life's simple pleasures, like holding hands and feeling sunshine on her face.
Nan inspires the best of human behavior in the people whom she meets.
There is a greater purpose for her survival. Her life has meaning and importance.

Wow. If you stop and think about it, these truths are pretty remarkable. In fact, they are awe-inspiring. When I read down this list I find it difficult to be negative. So I tuck it in the back of my mind so I can draw upon it when I feel my positive attitude beginning to waver.

Another powerful lesson I have learned is to choose my battles carefully. I no longer expend copious amounts of energy trying to mend things I know cannot be fixed. I only fight for what I know I can affect. I stay focused on my mission statement and use it as a compass to guide all my actions. It makes no sense to mourn that Nan has the disease. But I can make sure that she eats a healthy diet and exercises her brain on a daily basis to stave off her increasing symptoms.

A positive attitude ties back to the concept of accepting the reality of your loved one's situation and trying to make the most of where they are today. I am not telling you to put your head in the sand or overlook what is negative. I just want to encourage you to see every event in the best possible light.

The true test for me came when Nan fell and hurt her hip. Sadly she was never able to walk again. This was an emotionally devastating time for our entire family. Although her mental capabilities were rapidly declining, up until this point her physical health had remained strong. After hip surgery, her inability to walk proved not to be a physical problem, but instead was a consequence of her dementia. Although her legs were technically able to function, her brain was no longer sending nerve impulses down her spine commanding her leg muscles to tense and move. Consequently, she became permanently confined to a Geri-Chair.

You might be asking, "How could this be a good thing?" I know it sounds odd, but it actually was. Up until this time most of my worries centered on Nan's mobility. She was unsteady on her feet and fell quite frequently. She was inclined to wander and would often eat or come in contact with things that could harm her. Nan went through a long stage when she acted out physically and it was difficult to control her outbursts. She accosted workers or other residents who made her angry. Once she even wandered out into the middle of the street trying to find her way to our house. In those days every time the telephone rang I cringed and thought, "What now?"

My attitude may sound harsh, but Nan really did become safer once she was no longer able to walk. I could not modify her behavior by discussing my concerns. There was absolutely no reasoning with her. Every minute of every day, she was at risk. It became easier to manage her movements and keep her safe when she was no longer mobile. No one likes to think of someone they love being confined permanently to a wheelchair, but this instance is the exception. So you see what was a tragedy of sorts, was also a blessing. Family members of other dementia patients have told me that they were also relieved when their loved one became restricted to the safety of a wheelchair.

So instead of dwelling on what Nan was no longer able to do, the entire family embraced a positive approach. When we went to see her, we acted as though nothing had changed. Consequently, Nan was not distressed by the change in her condition. Before long she relaxed and completely accepted her new limitations. Now when we go outside for our walks, I use one hand to push the chair and the other to hold her hand. I truly believe that she thinks she is still walking right beside me. There are even times when she'll say to me, "Let's run!" In the end this seemingly major setback had a silver lining after all.

I urge you to not dwell on all that your loved one has lost or how things used to be. If you pay attention and look around, there is enough happiness left here, this very day, to help make up for all the losses they have endured. Embrace their limitations and find ways to convey joy in new and exciting ways, like holding hands while taking a stroll in a Geri-Chair. Finding solutions to difficult problems will steel your resolve and produce an often heady feeling of success. Don't count yesterday's blessings, count today's. For even with all the complications that you face, there remains much to be enjoyed in this moment. Let your optimism spill over into the life of your loved one.

No one can dispute that moods and feelings, both negative and positive, are contagious. We have all witnessed it. In my experience, dementia sufferers are particularly keen to respond to the verbal and nonverbal cues around them. Their thoughts are often so turbulent and difficult to decipher that they need you to help them gauge their surroundings. This means that you have to be very careful. If you are feeling particularly stressed or worried, take time to relax before you interact with your loved one.

Positive energy is the glue that holds the Moment by Moment technique together. In order to look past the sadness of dementia and truly believe that joy can be created in small moments, you have to be an optimist. When I speak of positivity I am referring to rational optimism as opposed to wishful thinking. The rational part of me knows that I can't cure or fix this situation. But the optimist that dwells in my heart believes that I possess the power to make Nan's disease tolerable, for her and for those around her. Optimists have the ability to step aside and look beyond themselves and their immediate needs. They are confident in the idea that things will be made right in the end and trust that they are on the right path. They acknowledge that their personal power can make a situation better.

When Nan hurt her hip and went to live in a nursing facility a doctor told me that she would be dead within six months. "Because she can no longer walk, she will frequently suffer from pneumonia. Although she may recover from the first few bouts, in the end it will take her. I don't think she will live longer than six months." This attitude shocked me. I realized that the doctor was just trying to be realistic, but I didn't appreciate this unhelpful and negative attitude. I explained to the doctor that although her prognosis may be statistically correct, she had not met my Nan and encountered her superwoman internal strength. I made it very clear that I was going to do everything possible to ensure that this did not happen. Needless to say, that was five years ago and my girl is still going strong.

It is important that you realize that you are the leader of your loved one's care team. You alone set the tone that instructs healthcare professionals how you want your loved one treated. You have the power to positively impact everyone who deals with your loved one—for example, doctors, caregivers, nurses, and other family members. By projecting a positive attitude, you relay the hopes that you have for your loved one's future. When I communicated my intentions to Nan's doctor, she walked away from our meeting knowing full well that I expected my mother-in-law to receive whatever care was necessary for her to live many years into the future. I was kind but firm when relaying my expectations. I also politely pulled her to the side and explained that I did not want negative health information or prognoses discussed in front of Nan.

Remember that you are the pacesetter, an ambassador of sorts. You are responsible for conveying your loved one's wishes and priorities to doctors, nurses, and other caregivers. In order to effectively build a working partnership with these professionals, you must face reality, look preparedly into the future, and motivate others to facilitate the physical and emotional goals that you have made for your loved one. A positive attitude creates synergy among the team and elicits future cooperation.

When I was young I loved reading *Reader's Digest*. Each month when it arrived I would sit and devour it. It contained stories on every topic imaginable and looking back, I learned many things by reading this small magazine. I have always remembered one particular piece. It was an article based on President Dwight D. Eisenhower's definition of leadership. He said, "Pull the string, and it will follow wherever you wish. Push it, and it will go nowhere at all."[1] This sentiment is apropos in all examples of leadership—even when leading a dementia care team. Make your intentions and expectations known to every professional from the very beginning. Begin as you mean to continue. Be clear and realistically optimistic. Ask for their help to obtain the goals you have for your loved one.

When dealing with anyone on the care team, always come from a place of gratitude. Speak of triumphs that were made possible because of their excellent care. If you do have a grievance, it will be better received if you sandwich it between two positive comments. State your concern simply to the appropriate individual and then follow up to ensure that the change has been made. Remember to give others a chance to rectify the situation. Most importantly keep in mind that their jobs are difficult and often thankless. Your goal should be to seek cooperation from every person trying to improve the life of your loved one. Remember, you want to pull your team along, not push it by constantly harping on negative scenarios and pointing out workers' failures. Keep the following points in mind when dealing with care workers:

- Empathy—Put yourself in the place of all those who are aiding you in this fight. Remember, there is no magic drug to stop this disease and caring for a dementia patient is both physically and mentally demanding.
- Respect—Practice the golden rule. Everyone in the team plays a vital role in the success of your plan. Treat them as you wish to be treated.
- Focus—Don't sweat the small stuff. Only address issues that directly impact the achievement of your mission statement.
- Clarity—Make your goals and expectations clear to everyone who is caring for your loved one. I have made it clear to the doctors and nursing staff that I want each day of Nan's life to be as joyful

as possible. No opportunity for happiness should be wasted or overlooked.

Over the years I have developed a dogged determination to remain positive about everything concerning Nan's dementia. But even though I can steer my thoughts in a positive direction, finding methods for elevating her self-esteem and positive energy have proven to be incredibly challenging. Dementia has completely robbed her of her confidence. She often tells me that she thinks that she is *stupid* or *crazy*. The only way I know to combat these thoughts is through constant reassurance and telling her positive stories from her life. I lavish her with encouraging feedback when she solves a simple problem or behaves in an appropriate manner. If she feeds herself an afternoon snack with no assistance, I compliment her dexterity. If she remembers the words to a song, I praise her strong memory. If she remembers what day it is, I tell her how happy I am that she is paying attention to the world around her. If she brushes her own hair, I tell her she has never looked lovelier. If you keep your eyes open, there are endless opportunities to offer kind praise and constructive reinforcement. Any task, no matter how small, can be turned into a positive interaction.

Sometimes when we are sitting together, I recount a list of her life achievements. I remind her of all that she has done for others, including me. I tell her that she is valuable and not to worry, we all become a bit confused at times. I explain how she has contributed to the happiness of my life. We talk about Homer Market and how she fed an entire town. I remind her of the many times that she took supplies to the inmates at the local jail, because, "There is good in everyone," and, "Not everyone gets a fair start in life." Sometimes she looks at me in wonder, like she is hearing these stories for the first time. But at the end, after she has learned that she is the heroine of my tale, her face beams with pride.

Decide today that you will face dementia with a positive attitude. Allow yourself to be elevated high above your immediate circumstances. Project enthusiasm in all you do for your loved one. Don't let negativity rob you of the best that life has to offer. Let no place be large enough to hold your optimism. Illuminate every life that comes in contact with you.

In the great book of life, each of us gets one page to fill. It is as white as magnolia blossoms, written with ink ground from sharp thorns mixed with sweet summer cherries. Its corners are dog-eared from the rereading of it. We are all continually writing our autobiography, word by word on these time-worn pages, until at last our letters become so faint that they predict our inevitable conclusion.

What is Nan writing during these final days of her life? As her pen slowly scratches forward, the letters are now too weak to make out and seem to be floating off into oblivion. But I hope she is writing of happy times even though her mind is fading. I hope she is writing of peace and tranquility as she prepares for her upcoming journey. And at the end when her last sentence is formed, I hope it will boldly proclaim that she has lived a life filled with wondrous surprises and abounding joy.

INSIGHTS

- Make a commitment each day to "just control the controllables." Make those twenty-four hours as enjoyable as possible for both your loved one and you.
- Only by adopting a positive attitude will you be able to participate and recognize the miracles that are swirling around your loved one.
- Fake it until you make it. Practice positive self-talk and life-affirming actions until they become a natural habit.
- You are the filter through which your loved one sees the world. If you are stressed and upset they will mimic your negative attitude. But if you are positive, you will remind them that love and hope are still possible.
- Celebrate your loved one's life. Make a list of all the positive circumstances surrounding their life and your role as a caregiver.
- Choose your battles carefully. Only fight for what you know you can affect. Don't waste energy trying to affect change that is not possible.
- Remember that you are the leader of your loved one's care team. You set the tone that conveys how your loved one should be treated emotionally and physically.
- Don't count yesterday's blessings, count today's.
- Remember to come from a place of thanks and gratitude when dealing with the team of individuals caring for your loved one.
- Stay focused on your mission statement.

6

MEMORIES

Memory is a child walking along a seashore. You never can tell what small pebble it will pick up and store away among its treasured things.

—Pierce Harris
Atlanta Journal

Dear Nan,

Today let's travel back to all the places you hold so dear. Let's leave the worries and confusion of the present behind. Together let's walk the dusty roads of your childhood, taking time to drink from the sweet springs of your youth. Let's time-travel to better days when you were whole. You lead the way and I will follow. Relax as the sun hits your face as you tend your garden. Rejoice as you join in the quiet contemplation of Sunday worship. Blush as you relive the day when you met your first sweetheart. Remind me of who you were. Tell me the stories of your life and through you, I will also remember.

We are the culmination of the memories that we collect throughout our lives. Whether good or bad, they are the origin of our beliefs and character. They are inescapable. Although we may not realize it, they foretell how we will interpret the world around us and set the tone for our close relationships. Our memories help us form instinctive responses to the situations and the people whom we encounter—a power so subtle that it often goes unnoticed.

During our lifetime each of us carries a battered trunk filled with scenes written on carefully preserved slips of paper, like the prophecies hidden inside fortune cookies. Our triumphs lay on top and are easily recalled: the day our child was born, the awards we won throughout our career, the time we broke the ribbon at the finish line as onlookers cheered. But quieter moments settle to the bottom and rarely cross our minds, like the first time we sank our feet into wet sand at the ocean's edge or heard our first Puccini aria.

Open your personal trunk and take a look inside. What do you see? Or better yet, who do you see? I see the faces of all those who loved me into being; some are now blurred by time like aging photos pasted in a worn picture album. I see the face of my first-grade teacher and the social worker who introduced me to my parents. I see the face of the man who offered me my first professional job and the face of my mother when she was singing Schubert.

But imagine who you would be today without all these images and memories from your past. Who would you be if they were suddenly stripped away, and when you looked into the face of your child a stranger was staring back at you?

Only when you have witnessed the "amnesia-ing" of a dementia patient, do you become fully aware of how memory loss changes the personality and character of an individual. All that we are is entangled within a web of our yesterdays, thread upon thread, until one is indistinguishable from the other. Our memories are the filters through which we interpret everything that happens in our lives. They help define our character and our passions. Without them our minds are homeless, separated forever from our identity.

I have spent an incalculable amount of time trying to imagine what it must be like to live inside Nan's world, existing in a reality filled with people and things that I do not recognize. What would it feel like to look in the mirror and not recognize your own face? What if right now you did not know where you were or how you got there? Imagine a stranger who you do not recognize trying to cajole you into submission in a soft patronizing tone. It must feel as if you and the world have gone mad. Is it any wonder that Nan is often fearful, argumentative, and combative?

Soon after Nan's diagnosis we began witnessing an obvious split between her short-term and her long-term memory. Since her moods, behaviors, and interpretation of reality are directly linked to both of these processes, at times you could almost see them working against each other.

As her short-term memory faded she became more confused about daily activities and everything in her surroundings. Trying to convince her of anything became almost impossible. I rarely made any headway and found myself refighting battles that I thought I had already won. I was constantly reintroducing her to the people caring for her and reminding her that she had moved to a new home. Eventually each visit began to feel like a scene from *Groundhog Day*.

What made things so complicated was that while her short-term memory was fading, her long-term memory remained in full operation. This meant that she still possessed a strong sense of *self* and outward confidence. She acted like the assured intelligent woman that she knew herself to be. She voiced her confused viewpoints with all the vigor of a campaigning politician and fought hard to drive home her singular interpretation of the world. Consequently, she was combative and difficult to manage. She was an absolute warrior in her attempt to prove that her mind was not muddled. No matter what the subject was, she fought hard to convince me that she was right and I was wrong. In truth I think she was trying to convince herself that she was still in control of her thoughts and her life. During this stage she was unwavering and stood her ground on even the tiniest matter. These were dark days filled with loud voices and attempted physical altercations on her part. I tried my best not to argue with her. After all, what was the point of quarreling with anyone in this condition? But she was armed and ready to go to battle with anyone who challenged her view of the world. Sometimes it felt like she fought just for the sake of fighting.

Then as if by magic, one day the war was over. Her short-term memory declined to such a point that she was forced to wave the white flag and surrender to her fate. She was unable to fight over the details of her life, because she could no longer remember them. She became remarkably calm. And then her long-term memory began to fill the gaps in her understanding. She began to focus more and more on her yesterdays, a time when life was less challenging and more recognizable.

This is not unusual. I have seen this happen to most of the dementia patients whom I have met. As the disease gains ground, recent events recede to the periphery of their thoughts and distant memories move forward to take their place. Biologically I know that there are scientific reasons why this occurs, but it also makes sense on an emotional level. The past is a safe haven of sorts, a place where they feel confident and secure. Instinctively they travel back to a time when they were in complete control of their mind and bodies. In a world that is uncertain and frankly scary, the sureness of the past becomes a comfortable and manageable place to dwell.

As dementia progresses, the schism between short- and long-term memory becomes increasingly wider and more difficult to bridge. This poses a dilemma for the caregiver who is trying to help the patient strike a balance between what happened long ago and what is happening in their world today. It is incredibly difficult to keep them based in reality in a way that will not cause arguments or feed their feelings of resentment. You can't simply tell them about their current situation and expect them to accept what you are saying as the truth. You can talk until you are blue in the face and never gain their cooperation. No, first you need to calm the situation and not let them see you as an enemy. You have to gain their trust by honoring this natural tendency to focus on the past.

The Moment by Moment technique encourages you to work from common ground, and the past is a good starting point. As I told you earlier, do not try to drag your loved one forward into your world. Instead join them where they are. Stop beating your head against the wall and take your cue from them. If you don't, you will feel like you are trying to go up a down escalator.

In Nan's case I set about finding ways to nurture both her short- and long-term memory. I accepted that her memory consists of two separate parts—her brief, often lightening quick, short-term memory and her distant memories from long ago. I accepted that these two thought processes are constantly at war with each other as she interprets what is going on around her. I accepted that one component of her memory is no more important than the other. On the contrary, each must be acknowledged in order to achieve the balance necessary to gain optimal cooperation and sustained happiness.

By honoring both her short- and long-term memory, I was better able to effectively manage her daily life and create positive interactions when we were together. I found ways to foster each one separately. This analytical approach to Nan's memory and cognitive decline empowered me. It made me less emotional and better equipped to deal with her inevitable outbursts and daily setbacks.

NURTURING SHORT-TERM MEMORY

The more we engage the dementia sufferer with the world around them, the more likely they are to remain an active participant in the present. Here are some suggestions for nurturing your loved one's short-term memory:

- Create and maintain a daily schedule. Healthy eating and sleeping habits are optimized when the patient is on a predetermined routine. The stress level of both the patient and caregiver decreases when a schedule is followed.

    There are distinct times of the day when it is necessary for a patient to be grounded in the present. These include the daily activities of normal living, like bathing, eating, sleeping, and taking medications. Typically many of these activities take place in the morning, but remember that this is not cast in stone. Nan happens to be at her best in the morning so I schedule her doctors' appointments or nurses' visits for these hours. But if this is not the case for your loved one, be flexible. If they are more amiable after lunch, schedule their showers in the afternoon or at bedtime. Remember that you need to be the one to adjust and become attuned to their natural rhythms. Do not force them to follow some predetermined or arbitrary schedule or routine.
- Hang a whiteboard in your loved one's main living area. Write the current day of the week and date along with any activities that are scheduled for that day. Include a list of telephone numbers and emergency contacts. This is helpful if they are still able to use a telephone, but it also provides caregivers quick access to contact numbers in case of emergency.
- Don't allow your loved one to spend the entire day in one room. Remaining in one spot all day makes it difficult to detect the passage of time and increases the likelihood that they will sleep during daylight hours and be awake at night. In order to maintain healthy sleep habits, bedrooms should, if at all possible, be

designated for naps and nighttime sleeping. Staying in one room all day can also create feelings of isolation. When disconnected from the outside world, the dementia patient is more likely to suffer from confusion and depression.

- Encourage your loved one to interact with the people in the world around them. Caregivers, visitors, and other patients are a wonderful source of companionship for the dementia patient. Again, the more they feel a part of the world around them, the more likely they are to remain in it. Yes, I know there are biological events occurring that are fighting against this, but I am a firm believer in the "use it or you lose it" philosophy. Engaging in relationships outside of their immediate family circle increases feelings of independence and helps rebuild confidence.

- Keep your loved one informed about the world around them. Discuss positive current events within your family and the world. By asking their opinion on a variety of subjects, you force them to concentrate and communicate their beliefs. It also helps remind them that they are a part of something larger than themselves.

- Remember to be positive. Offer praise and positive reinforcement when your loved one remembers an event, solves a problem, or recalls information that you have relayed to them. This will increase their confidence and help combat the fear that they are going crazy.

NURTURING LONG-TERM MEMORY

As a caregiver it may seem counterintuitive to nurture their long-term memory. After all that is where they spend most of their time. You may ask, "Why bother? It seems like I spend all of my time trying to get them to remember things in the short-term. As it is, they only talk about events that happened decades ago."

In the beginning I subscribed to this idea and worked vigilantly to correct the lapses in Nan's short-term memory. I was determined to drag her forward into the present. Unfortunately, this approach never created common ground or built a link between our two worlds.

Keep your eye on the prize and remember your mission statement. You cannot create experiences that bring peace and joy into their lives if you are constantly trying to make them remember information or perform tasks. This avenue will never lead to happiness, let alone cooperation.

So I decided to join Nan and spend time with her inside her memories. Some of our most tender and poignant times together have been spent reliving her past. Our relationship and mutual fellowship grew each day because she knew that I truly wanted to hear what she had to say. When I heard her stories I validated her feelings and honored who she is as a person. Granted, like *Cliffs Notes* they lacked detail. I spent a lot of my time trying to fill in the missing scenes or characters, but somehow in the end I was able to understand. By cherishing scenes from Nan's past, I have come to understand and know her on a deeper level. Even through the fog of confusion she managed to share the milestones of her life with me. I am privileged to be able to carry her stories forward. They emboldened me to keep pushing onward in my attempt to build her a better life.

But sadly time marches on, and unfortunately so does dementia. Eventually it robbed me of these special moments. Nan no longer remembers the details of her past or the names of those whom she has loved so dearly. This is all the more reason to make use of the time you have today and listen to what your loved one has to say. Tuck their stories away in your trunk of memories for the day when you will become the storyteller who retells the tales of their life.

I encourage you to embrace the idea of nourishing your loved one's long-term memory. Offer them a respite from their feelings of inadequacy and frustration. Let them have a safe refuge where they can rest and be calm. Encourage them to remember who they once were and all that they represent. And who knows, you might even share a laugh or two.

- Set aside time during the day to sit quietly and ask your loved one questions about their past. I found that after one or two questions Nan was off and running, busily describing the events of a past adventure. If they get the details wrong, don't correct them. It is more important that they express their feelings than be accurate. If sad memories arise, redirect the conversation by asking questions on a new and more positive topic.

- Create a *Memories Board* to hang in their main living space. Purchase a large bulletin board and cover the background with colorful wrapping or craft paper. Then, using your computer, print in large bold letters the title or theme of your board. For Nan's board I printed *Nan's Wonderful Life* and positioned it along the top edge. Next, scan and print pictures that represent the most important people and events of their life.

   Be selective. The idea is not to cover the entire board with photographs. Remember, too much information can confuse a dementia patient. Leave space between the pictures. If you like, you can print captions to coincide with each photograph in order to help jog their memory. Not only does this help your loved one, but it also offers caregivers a glimpse into the life of their patient. It becomes a way for the aides to gain an in-depth understanding of the unique individual in their care.

- Create a photo album filled with pictures of the patient's loved ones from the past and present. This is a wonderful catalyst for conversation when you visit and they can enjoy the album when they are alone. Be sure to label each picture to help prompt their recollections. Nan loves looking through her album, and I cannot overstate what a wonderful source of comfort it has been for her. I have even been told by facility workers that she often carries it around with her throughout the day.

Set out to do everything in your power to keep your loved one engaged with the world around them, but don't underestimate the peace and tranquility that can be gained by allowing them to ramble through their past. Help them find ways to cope with their two separating worlds. Remember that like you and me, their memories define their existence. Let them float above their worries from time to time and remember better days. Facilitate their journey with your patience and love. Listen to their stories and let their experiences live on within you.

Act now because time is ticking on. Soon that battered trunk will slip slowly from their fingers, falling open as it hits the ground, and all you will be able to do is try to catch those small slips of paper before the wind carries them off into oblivion.

INSIGHTS

- Work hard to nurture both the long-term and short-term memory of your loved one.
- Do not try to quell the dementia patient's desire to relive their yesterdays. Instead join them and stroll down memory lane together. Let them tell you the stories of their life.
- Utilize their long-term memories in order to evoke feelings of happiness and pride.
- Reinforce your loved one's short-term memory by creating a daily schedule, encouraging them to interact with the people around them, and schedule important activities for the time of day when they are most alert and convivial.
- Create a *Memories Board* to hang in their room and create a photo album recounting the people and events of their wonderful life.
- If your loved one becomes sad when speaking of a specific memory, acknowledge their feelings and then redirect the conversation toward happier topics.

7

BEAUTY

We live in a wonderful world that is full of beauty, charm and adventure. There is no end to the adventures that we can have if only we seek them with our eyes open.

—Jawaharlal Nehru

We are what we see. We are products of our surroundings.

—Amber Valletta

There is a legend that one night while St. Francis was strolling through his beloved Assisi, he watched a brilliant silvery moon rise high in the night sky. Bewitched by this pale jewel set against midnight's soft velvet, he decided that this magnificent beauty should be witnessed by the entire world. So he ran to the church bell tower and began to ring the bells, with no regard to the late hour or the danger these chimes usually foretold. He kept ringing the bells until all the weary town's people had gathered around the church below. When asked what evil threatened their town, St. Francis stretched out his arms and said, "Lift up your eyes, my friends. Look at the beauty of the moon!"

Beauty, even with all of her subjective implications, is a profound and powerful muse. She spreads a blanket of loveliness at our feet, so we do not have to feel life's harsh rocks embedded in the earth beneath us. She is the cloak that protects us against the biting sleet that cuts our skin and stings our eyes. She is quiet tranquility in a world filled with ringing phones and car horns, a buffer, a cushion on which to lay our weary heads so that we can dream of better days. Beauty elevates us so that we can peer over the mountain top and witness the serenity of a green and distant valley. Beauty changes us; it changes everything. This ancient Chinese proverb says it best: "When you have only two pennies left in the world, buy a loaf of bread with one, and a lily with the other."

Years ago I managed an interior design firm that had a clientele of wonderfully eccentric wealthy customers. *Designing Women* was a popular television show at this time, and we were constantly asked if our work life mirrored the scenes from the show. Yes, the business office was in an old mansion, and we did sit in a beautiful living room surrounded by antiques, but that was where the similarities stopped. We were conducting business, not dishing out the details of our personal lives.

By being invited into clients' secret worlds, this job opened my eyes to how people live inside their private spaces. One particular client stands out among the rest. When I first met her, she seemed sad and, frankly, depressed. Her demeanor appeared downtrodden and she hired our firm at her husband's insistence. When we made our initial visit to her home we were shocked. The walls in her living space were black, not dark gray or green, but jet-black. No wonder her partner demanded that she hire a team of designers to change her home's interior.

In the course of the next few months, we transformed her residence from a dark gothic dungeon into a stylish sophisticated home. But most surprising was the change that we saw in her. As her home was revitalized, her mood seemed to change. As her walls and furnishings became brighter, her attitude seemed more positive. Unknowingly we had provided our own dose of antidepressants in the form of paint, fabric, and furniture. Of course her beautiful new environment could not solve all her problems, but at least she now lived in an uplifting and enriching home. And who knows? We might have even saved a marriage.

During my tenure, I witnessed countless versions of this story that prove that our physical home environment can directly influence our overall sense of happiness and well-being. The setting in which we spend our time impacts our attitudes and affects how we see ourselves in the world. It impacts our productivity and contentment. This knowledge is a powerful tool that, if utilized properly, can elevate our moods and bring peace into our lives. Living in a beautiful and organized environment reduces our stress, feeds our spirit, and makes room for all of life's possibilities.

If you have spent any time at all in an assisted living or nursing facility, you know that these institutions have had to sacrifice beauty for the sake of functionality. They tend to feel cold and uninviting—certainly not a place that anyone would choose to call home. I find this remarkable and frankly, a bit sad. Just because someone has fallen ill or is no longer able to live alone does not lessen the positive impact that a beautiful environment can have on their life. On the contrary. In this instance, the power of beauty with all its benefits is even more necessary.

Typically when I walk down the halls of Nan's nursing facility, I peer into many rooms that are dark and lonely. Even on a beautiful sunny day the curtains will be closed so tightly that they shut out even the smallest chink of light. And there the patient lies alone in a room lit only by the blue electronic glow of a television set. No wonder nursing home patients frequently mix up their days and nights. Who wouldn't? How can anyone maintain their will to live, or get well for that matter, in such a dismal and depressing environment? When I see this, it takes all my control not to march into these rooms, fling open the curtains, and hunt for a bit of Mozart on the radio.

No matter what our circumstances or where we live, we need to experience the essentials of life in order to keep our minds and souls active and vibrant. We must be exposed to adequate light, fresh air, sunshine, and beauty. And the elderly, sick, and memory impaired are no exception. To ignore this fact is to rob them of their humanity.

Whether your loved one lives in a facility or in a room in your home, it makes no difference; the same fundamental principles apply. A clean, bright, and beautiful environment will impact how they feel about themselves and their situation. As caregivers, we should keep in mind how environment can positively impact the lives of the dementia sufferer. Our challenge is to take an ordinary or institutional environment and make it pleasurable and beautiful. I am not suggesting that you spend a great deal of money. So many stylish and lovely home products are available at reasonable prices online and in discount stores. Keep in mind, you will also be spending a great deal of time in this room, so why not make it lovely for both of you?

LIGHT

Optimal lighting is possibly the most important design element when creating a safe and cheerful environment for the dementia sufferer. It is as vital as fresh air and nutritious food. If utilized correctly it can uplift their mood and impact their body rhythms. Light, or the absence of light, sets the tone for all that occurs within a space and fosters optimal mental health. Nothing beautiful can be appreciated in a room that is dark and dingy. Good lighting clarifies, inspires, and illuminates our surroundings, while bad lighting can make us weary, confused, or overly stimulated.

Consider the following three points when evaluating the lighting in your loved one's environment. First, an impaired person who lives in a well-lit environment is less likely to fall or stumble. Second, since many dementia patients suffer from paranoia, illuminating dark areas and hallways evokes a feeling of reassurance and safety. And third, bright and adequate lighting can elevate moods and help regulate sleep and eating patterns. Our goal should be to combine the beauty found in proper lighting with the natural healing properties that it contains.

As we age, the necessity for adequate light exposure increasingly plays a key role in our overall health. The correlation between light and well-being becomes even more important for a patient diagnosed with dementia. Due to the symptomatic changes that occur as a result of the disease, it is imperative that patients be exposed to adequate amounts of bright light in order to maintain the body's natural circadian rhythm. This rhythm controls the biological events that are repeated every twenty-four hours. When this rhythm is disturbed or out of sync, it can cause depression, sleep disturbances, and decreased appetites.[1] Studies have also concluded that residents living in care facilities with low light levels are more likely to suffer from high agitation and anxiety.[2]

Therefore, the first and most important step to creating a healthy and beautiful environment for your loved one is to evaluate the lighting in their current living space. If your loved one lives in a facility, you probably visit during daylight hours and rarely see their surroundings in the evening or at twilight. I suggest that you pay a visit at dusk and make sure their room feels bright and cheerful. Do not hesitate to add additional lamps to make the room feel safe and cozy. You will be surprised what two good lamps can do to enrich the atmosphere and diminish the sterile feeling of an institution.

Overwhelming scientific evidence demonstrates that exposure to light on the skin or through the eyes affects mental as well as physical health. No light source on the market will replace our innate need for natural sunlight. However, when a patient is ill or forced to spend most of their time indoors, problems can arise. Research tells us that prolonged exposure to distorted spectrum light from fluorescent bulbs has a profound effect on an individual's mental outlook, moods, agitation levels, and general health.[3] So I suggest that you purchase a bit of sunshine. There are full-spectrum and daylight-spectrum light bulbs available on the market today that produce light that mimics the wavelengths that occur in sunlight.

The fluorescent light that was originally installed above Nan's bed gave the room a kind of a sad purplish glow, so I asked her facility if I could replace it with a full-spectrum bulb. Additionally, I placed similar bulbs in the lamps on her bedside table and on her dresser. Although traditional incandescent bulbs offer a warm glow, they project light from the red portion of the spectrum that does not duplicate the properties found in natural light.

Don't be cheap. On dark days and in the early evening, turn on the lights. I have made it clear to Nan's care team that I want her lights to be turned on at dusk and only turned off when it is time for her to sleep. If this is not feasible, connect your loved one's lamps to automatic timers so that you can control what time of day they will be turned on and off. The atmosphere and visual comfort that good lighting provides cannot be overstated. Brighten their world and their mood by turning on the lights!

COLOR

The science of color is utilized to impact our behaviors in all aspects of our everyday life. Although somewhat subjective, the basic effects of color have a universal meaning.[4] If you don't believe me, ask yourself these questions: Why is bread packaging typically red? Why are doctors' offices typically painted a calming shade of blue or green? Why is bright pink the preferred color for drunk tank walls? Why do delivery drivers wear brown? Why is orange found throughout do-it-yourself home stores? Why is silver the color associated with wealth management? None of this happens by coincidence. No, these colors were put in place to directly affect our behavior.

Ancient cultures including those of the Egyptians and the Chinese practiced chromotherapy, or the use of color to aid in healing.[5] This practice is still utilized today in alternative and holistic health treatments. I suggest that you keep this in mind when selecting paint colors for your loved one's environment. Choose a color that will not only enhance their mood, but will also evoke a feeling of home and safety. This is particularly important when they are in the early stages of dementia and are still fully engaged in their immediate surroundings. For the cost of a few gallons of paint, you can create a peaceful and soothing environment.

Take time to reflect on your loved one's preferences. What is their favorite color? Or for that matter, what colors do they dislike? What colors were predominant in their previous home? I have found that most assisted living facilities will allow you to paint a resident's room; just be sure to have the color pre-approved. This may not be possible in a nursing home situation, so you'll have to be a bit more creative. Consider using color therapy when selecting your loved one's bedspread, window curtains, and blankets.

As we have learned from my client with the black walls, the color of our living environment tremendously impacts how we feel about ourselves and our situation. Color leaves an impression and can positively or negatively affect our attitude. Think of color as a kind of mood prescription, a tool that if utilized effectively can help create an atmosphere of peace and well-being.

When Nan moved into her assisted living facility, we were lucky. The previous resident had painted the walls a soft and soothing shade of blue. At the time Nan was going through a stage of heightened agitation, so blue was the perfect color for her environment because it evokes a feeling of calm and tranquility.

Before you make a final decision, consider how we emotionally react to the following colors:

- Red tends to stimulate the body and mind. It has even been suggested that looking at the color red can increase your pulse, heart rate, and blood pressure.
- Yellow is a sunny color and evokes happiness and sunshine. However, if not used in moderation, it can cause excitement.
- Blue is proven to add comfort to an environment and is even helpful for the treatment of pain. It also creates a calm, relaxed, and serene setting.
- Green is both restful and refreshing. It mimics the restorative powers found in nature.
- Pink is joyful and romantic. People in pink spaces tend to become calmer. This so called "pink effect" even seems to continue for twenty minutes after leaving the room.
- White walls can feel airy and spacious, but can also feel bland, cold, and institutional.[6]

Whatever color you end up selecting, it is important to keep your color hues soft. Intense or bright versions of any color could make the patient anxious and uncomfortable. Soft blue was perfect for Nan, where as a bright vibrant blue would not have achieved the same effect. If your loved one likes warm colors like yellow, consider matching the color of freshly churned butter. Remember we want to create a soothing environment. So even if they love bright red, instead of using it on the walls or furniture, use it as an accent color or a pillow for their chair.

FURNISHINGS

Now that you have decided on the best color for the backdrop and the stage is well lit, it is time to get started on the best part, the props.

When it becomes necessary for your loved to leave home and move into a more protective environment, you will want to be very discerning when selecting the furniture that will fill their new home. Unless they have priceless antiques or extremely valuable furniture, you will probably be able to create a lovely living environment with furnishings that they already own. In Nan's case we made it a point to incorporate a few of her favorite pieces so that she would have a feeling of familiarity with her environment. We kept the same bed that she slept in throughout her marriage but protected it with a plastic mattress cover. Next we moved in two comfortable reclining chairs, one for her and one for visitors. This ensured that she had a comfortable place to relax and watch television, listen to music, or talk on the telephone. A recliner was an excellent choice, since there were nights when it was necessary for one of us to stay with her due to illness or behavioral issues. I placed them next to a bright window and gave each its own side table and lamp. Next I purchased a small shelving unit so that she had a place for her CD player and family photographs. And lastly, I included a small wooden chair from the farm that I placed in the corner for the times when she had multiple visitors.

Make sure that all your loved one's soft furnishings are machine washable. This includes curtains, bedspreads, pillow covers, slipcovers, and shower curtains. Keep in mind that as their dementia progresses, their coordination will become impaired, making it more likely that they will spill food and drinks. So plan ahead and prepare now, because you will want to be able to take everything home and give it a good wash from time to time.

At this point you may be asking, "What does all this have to do with beauty?" My answer is, "Everything." By making correct and conscious choices, you can create an environment that specifically reflects the personality of your loved one. You can let your creativity take over. In Nan's case, I found some beautiful cotton fabric that had the look of old English chintz. Its ivory background and flowers in soft blue, yellow, pink, and green were a cheerful addition to her room. I made her curtains, throw pillows, and shams for her bed. I then purchased a butter yellow bedspread and found inexpensive, machine washable, soft blue slipcovers online for her recliners. I added a few new white lamp-shades with bright, full-spectrum bulbs and her studio room looked fresh, happy, and beautiful.

My goal was to create a home for Nan that was safe and functional, but also beautiful, and I think I succeeded. I chose everything deliber-ately to ensure efficiency and practicality. Here are some ideas worth considering:

- Eliminate all throw rugs or obstacles that could cause your loved one to trip and fall.

- If their furniture has sharp edges, consider covering them with insulation foam or childproof corner covers that can be found at any hardware store.
- Attach their television remote control to the table leg near their chair using plastic cinch ties and a curling expandable cord. This way the remote can be easily found and is less likely to be accidentally thrown away.
- Remove all mirrors from their environment so that reflected images do not confuse or scare them.
- Do not hang framed artwork in high traffic areas such as hallways, where they can easily fall and cause injury.
- If given the choice, always choose plastic instead of glass for objects in their environment—even in photo frames.
- Hang a large, easy-to-read clock on the wall opposite their favorite chair. Many digital clocks even display a.m. and p.m. I found this helpful when Nan began confusing her days and nights.

SIMPLICITY

When selecting objects for your loved one's environment, it is essential that you keep things simple. Choose only the items that you are certain will enhance their existence. Use a discerning eye when making your selections. To a mind that is already whirling with confusion, clutter only exacerbates the situation. Remember: your goal is to create a calm and peaceful haven that will provide them a place to relax and be still. Too many possessions can become irrationally worrisome for the dementia sufferer who may feel that they need to protect and care for each object. Take the Zen approach by engaging in the act of unselecting. Once you have collected all the items that you feel are necessary, edit them once again. Pare down your choices in order to keep things as simple as possible.

I learned this the hard way. Even though I tried to implement this plan, my first attempts at simplicity were a complete failure. When Nan moved into her assisted living facility I wanted her world to feel cozy and inviting, so I moved some of her treasures into her new apartment. Soon it became clear that I had really missed the mark. Since the onset of her disease, items that were once her treasures began to overstimulate her mind to the point of distraction. One afternoon when I came to visit I found most of her possessions lying in a pile outside of her door. She had taken it upon herself to remedy the situation by removing the clutter from her environment. Yet again, Nan had provided me with insight into her present condition and put me back on track. After her big clear-out, all that remained were photos of people she loved and a few small figurines that I had bought for her at the dollar store. Sadly, my magpie had long since flown away.

Don't ever assume that dementia patients or those relegated to the confines of a nursing facility no longer have a place in their lives for beauty. Even though the disease continues to ravage their mind, we can still elevate their spirit by introducing beauty into their everyday life. Take every opportunity to lavish their lives with loveliness. Point out beauty everywhere you see it. Whether in a child's face, a budding flower in a charming vase, or a sky streaked with fire at sunset, reconnect them to the wonders of the physical beauty in their life.

Let beauty be the poetry that sooths their soul. Let it be the salt that season's every aspect of their daily existence, the paper on which their dreams are writ. Let it remind them of what it means to be alive.

INSIGHTS

- The environment in which we live can directly impact our emotional moods and attitudes.
- Do not overlook the power that beauty has to create positive feelings when creating an environment for your loved one.
- Remember that even though your loved one is suffering from dementia, they still respond to basic human comforts like light, fresh air, sunshine, and beauty.
- Take a Zen approach when creating beauty in your loved one's environment. Remove all inhibiting and distracting possessions.
- Recognize that as we age, our need for adequate light exposure increases. Light your loved one's world to help ensure their safety and mental health.
- If your loved one is living in a nursing home, replace traditional fluorescent light bulbs with full-spectrum alternatives. If your loved

one is living at home, replace traditional incandescent light bulbs with full-spectrum bulbs.

- Carefully select the color of your loved one's main living space. Choose a tone that will encourage peace and tranquility.
- Consider functionality and familiarity when selecting furniture for their environment.
- Make sure that all your loved one's soft furnishings are machine washable.
- Eliminate clutter from their environment. If too many objects are in their surroundings they could feel overwhelmed and confused.

8

CREATING EMOTIONAL MEMORIES

Live because the sun falls in glimpses through leaves. Live because
the cold sends goosebumps down your skin. Live because it rains.
Live because the rainbows shine.

—Geeta Masurekar[1]

Toward the end of his life, Marcel Proust returned home one cold
afternoon feeling melancholic and chilled to the bone. Although not
typically a tea drinker, he agreed to join his mother for a warming cup
to help sooth his body and spirit. On this particular day his mother
served a plate of small delicious sponge cake cookies called *petit
madeleines*. He dunked a small piece of the delicate cookie into his tea.
Suddenly he was transported back in time to a Sunday morning at his
childhood home in Combray, France. Two moments of his life had
unexpectedly merged into one. There before him, as if in a play, was his
village, his neighbors, their homes, the parish church, Monsieur Swan's
garden, and all of sweet Combray. Only he and his aunt were home on
this remembered Sunday, since neither had gone to morning Mass.
When the young Marcel stopped by her room to wish her good day, he
was offered a taste of her madeleine cookie soaked in lime-blossom tea.
And now the taste of this same cookie many years later evoked one
exquisite moment of remembering. Soon after this, Marcel took to his
bed and began writing his thousand-page memoir entitled *Remembrance of Things Past*. It is hard to believe that the largest and most
illustrious work of his life was derived from a simple cup of tea enjoyed
on a cold winter's day.

Like Marcel, each of us has experienced a similar unexpected re-membering at some time in our life. When an old song that you have not heard in years plays on the radio, you are immediately catapulted back to a Friday night sock-hop in your high school gymnasium. Or one passing whiff of your deceased mother's perfume, and you are young again, sitting cross-legged on her bed, watching her prepare for a night out with your father. When she gets up to leave, she sprays a bit on the inside of your wrist and her scent lingers long after the babysitter has put you to bed. Or like dear Marcel, you might taste a memory, like the elephant ear pastry you ate one hot summer evening at the county fair. It reminds you of ancient carnival dust and that metallic smell that lingers on your hands after gripping the guard rail of the roller coaster.

Involuntary memories cast powerful spells, offering glimpses of a previous scene or moment in our lives. For that one instant, we become time travelers moving backward through the ripples of our lives, reliv-ing the loveliness of our yesterdays. When it happens we freeze, re-maining still, trying to recapture all the sensations in that one single moment. Like an archaeologist who spots one small shard of clay pot-tery poking up through the topsoil, we mentally excavate, digging deep-er, until we uncover whatever recollections surround this memory. It's déjà vu of sorts, only better, because these are memories that belong to us and not ghosts that we do not recall. Magic happens in these mo-ments that tear down the thin sheet of rice paper that separates us from our past. These unexpected incidents connect us with who we once were, our yesterdays. They have great power to bring us joy. They remind us of the continuum of our lives.

I wanted to awaken Nan to these small instruments of memory. I wanted to help her remember the previous chapters of her own story. So I became an investigator searching for clues in her distant past. I worked to learn as much as I could about her old life. I searched for even the smallest occurrence that might re-create those magical experi-ences. Granted, I really had no idea what she would respond to and doubted if I would be able to measure my success. But nothing was going to stop me from trying to uncover her triggers. Is it the smell of Ivory soap that she used to bathe her babies? Or the smell of gardenia blossoms like those she carried on her wedding day? Or the smell of the ocean when she strolled along the boardwalk in Virginia Beach during her days in the Navy? Or the cologne worn by an unknown beau from long ago? These aides-mémoire are so personal and subtle, they can be difficult to define. All I could do was to think back to a time before the unraveling began, to the days when all the choices of the world still lay at her feet, when she was in charge of her own life—back to the days when I first met her, back to her beloved farm.

The front room of Nan's farmhouse looked out onto the neighbor's soybean fields, which lay just past the swinging garden gate, beyond a large, silver mailbox and across a dusty country road. Her picture window with its nineteenth-century molding framed this idyllic country scene in each season as it turned. The room was neat and tidy with every treasure placed atop a lace doily that protected her waxed wood surfaces. And it smelled lovely, like a bouquet of freshly picked flowers, ladylike and sweet, just like Nan. She loved Crabtree and Evelyn's Spring Rain scent for both her body and her house. So this is where I began. I'd decided to scent her and her rooms in this dainty familiar fragrance.

I knew from my years of gift giving that this scent was available in a variety of products, so I set about building my stockpile. I purchased everything from room sprays to body lotion to draw liners. If it came in the Spring Rain fragrance, I bought it. And thankfully, I had been right. From the first dab of cologne placed on her inside wrist, I was certain that she had made the connection. She began to smile and then, as if to close off all her other senses, she closed her eyes and inhaled deeply. She had recognized it. Whether it transported her back to her cozy farmhouse, I can never be certain. But I truly believe that for that one short instant, I had tapped into something deep and secret, a private sensory memory that transported her back to happier days.

Then I turned my attention to music. Even though I knew that she loved her Baptist hymns, this wasn't the effect I was going for. I was trying to conjure the romance and excitement of her youth. As any baby boomer knows, when our parents were young they danced to the music synonymous with World War II and the Big Band Era. So I bought a boxed set of Glenn Miller's greatest hits from the late 1930s and 1940s. Although I am no expert on the music from these decades, I did recognize a few songs like "Moonlight Serenade," "Don't Sit under the Apple Tree," and "Tuxedo Junction." I began with "Chattanooga Choo Choo," which made her smile and say, "Oh, my." Before the second verse began she was tapping her foot to the beat of the music.

Did I call forth some memory thought to be lost forever? With dementia, you can never be certain. All I know is that I made her happy and filled a few minutes of her life with joy. After all, that is the whole idea. Since then we have enjoyed many happy hours listening to these uplifting hits. And anyway, how do I know that when she is smiling and tapping her feet, she is not jitterbugging across some USO dance floor with a handsome Petty Officer just before he ships out? As Shakespeare's Hamlet so perfectly put it, "There's the rub."[2] I will never know. I am searching for proof that does not exist.

We humans are needy by nature. We want to see the results of our labors, right now, this very minute. We want to witness hard evidence and calculate measurable results so that we can track our accomplishments. We want to know that we are making a difference and if so, by how much. Unfortunately, I must warn you that if you want constant evidence that you are getting through to an individual who suffers from dementia, you will end up feeling defeated and a bit crazy. I'm sorry, but dementia doesn't work like that. You have to tally your efforts the same as you would your known successes. You have to give yourself credit for each time you answer the call "Batter-up" and swing at the ball, not just when you round third and slide into home plate.

There is an interesting memory phenomenon that I have witnessed not only with Nan, but also with other dementia patients. Over time I began to see a correlation between how often I came to see Nan and her tendency to act out in a negative manner. The more often I came, the less likely she was to be anxious and distressed. It took some time for me to notice the pattern and to link these two events together. This is especially interesting since more often than not, she completely forgets my visit before I reach my car in the parking lot. So I am not saying that she remembers the actual details of our time together, but on some deeper level she seems to understand that someone loves and cares for her. It is as if a part of her knows that I have been to see her and this deeper connection seems to sustain her while I am away.

Research shows that Nan is not alone in this phenomenon. Experts have witnessed this also. According to research "endorphins released during a pleasant experience have a salutary effect on the person with dementia even after the experience is forgotten."[3]

After watching Nan for many years, I know with certainty that her understanding of the world around her is far greater than she is able to consciously recall or verbally communicate. It is as if her memory has been divided into two sections. The side of her mind that rationalizes and problem solves is being devoured by the ravages of her disease. It is worldly and temporal, directly affecting her ability to reason and problem solve. But then there is another side that relates to feelings of her heart. Although affected, it still seems able to respond to and retain loving experiences. For example, the more often I visit, the less likely she is to be aggressive and have emotional outbursts. She tends to be calmer, less agitated, and more cooperative. I don't know if it is conscious or intuitive, but I am absolutely certain that she knows on some level when I have been to see her and when I have not.

I am a realist. I know that Nan no longer can recount the details of our conversations or what time I said I'd return. But all the same, I know that my daily visits are not in vain. For when I have been absent for just one day, she clearly makes her feelings known. You would be amazed to see how a woman, who rarely speaks and on most days does not know her last name, will become angry with me because I was not at lunch on the previous day.

And boy, do I pay a heavy price when this happens. You might say that she and I become the Abbott and Costello of the nursing home circuit. We have our comedy routine down pat. Each of us knows our part and we perform it for the entertainment of the nursing home staff. We are a cross between a dreadful improvisation and an old tired comedy sketch that has earned lukewarm reviews along the vaudeville circuit.

It goes something like this: As I am walking down the hall, I see her and we lock eyes. I smile and wave. I receive a stony stare in response. At this point, I know that I am in big trouble. My first impulse is to turn, jump in my car, and hightail it out of there, but I know from experience that I would only be postponing the inevitable. It is best to take my lickings and get it over with. As I approach her Geri-Chair she puts her hand up so I can't kiss her and then jerks her head to the side so that she doesn't have to look at me. I respond by acting as if nothing is wrong. I ask her how she is feeling and if she is getting hungry. If my intuition tells me that things are looking particularly bleak, I pull out all the stops and tell her how lovely she looks. At this point two possible things can happen. I will either be given her *evil eye* or be verbally assaulted by the worst possible names she can call to mind. Two of my favorites are *Dummy* and *Meanie*, which never fail to bring the house down. Although the nurses try to politely cough so I won't hear their laughter, I know that if given the opportunity they would stomp their feet, flick their lighters and cheer with delight. Yes, I know, "Sticks and stones . . ."And anyway, who am I to deny a little afternoon entertainment to these hardworking people?

Next Nan gives me what I like to call her *shriveler*. This expression looks something like this: She tilts her head to one side, shuts her eyes, puts her nose in the air and absolutely refuses to look at me. I try to get her to respond, much like a mother who is trying to get her toddler to smile for the camera. But no amount of cajoling works. She is nothing if not determined. If she has a mind to, she can continue this attitude with the endurance of any Olympic athlete. Of course, this makes feeding her lunch a bit tricky, since the side of her head is facing me. If I move myself in front of her face, she will just change the direction of her *shriveler*, and once again I am trying to put food in her mouth at a right angle.

I don't want to leave you with the impression that she is in any way crabby or unkind. In fact, she is quite the contrary. As if to prove her disdain for me and drive her point home, she will smile and wave to everyone in her proximity, like a queen sitting in a jewel-encrusted Geri-Coach. Oh no, she saves her *shriveler* for me alone, her lowly private livery.

I tell you this story because I am trying to encourage you to not be shortsighted and to never discount your loved one's level of understanding. It is impossible for us, no matter how well we think we know them, to completely understand what makes its way through their mental clutter. I find it amazing that even in the late stages of her disease, Nan is still able to unleash this effective form of emotional blackmail. I say blackmail, because it works every time. I am easy prey and she knows it. I leave feeling as if I have let her down and vowing to myself that I won't miss another day. Chalk one up to Miss Nan.

If you think that this is completely farfetched, observe your loved one after you have been absent for a day or two. Although they might not be as aggressively punitive as Nan, I bet that if you pay attention you will see a change in their attitude toward you. Be thankful and take this as a sign of hope. After all, it proves what you and I have known all along—that they are still in there.

I truly believe that the spirit of every interaction, every smile, every loving comment, and every joy-filled instant, stays with Nan deep inside her spirit. Consequently, I do not discount any positive interaction that she and I have. I believe in the encouraging impact of regular loving contact.

Unfortunately, as I stated earlier, most of your progress will not be obvious. Most of the time, it will be invisible. For you see, you can never know what is remembered deep within your loved one's heart. Just because you cannot see a reaction to the efforts that you make, do them anyway. Just because you cannot guarantee that they will remember that they are loved, love them anyway. For, if you count your successes by visible affirmations you will surely be disappointed.

No, your rewards will be paid to you in the best currency of all, in the knowledge that you and your loved one have experienced tiny pleasures that otherwise may have gone unnoticed. Sometimes these pleasures will seem so small that you will wonder if they were worth your bother. Oh, but they were. Begin collecting them today. Pick them up joy-by-joy, pebble-by-pebble, until there are no stones of happiness left on the beach to be wasted and washed back into the sea.

Honor the person who still lives deep inside your loved one. Even though they are burrowed far beneath their conscious connections, call forth sensory memories from their life by reintroducing them to things that they once loved. Remember that you, as their caregiver, have the ability to positively inject happiness into their spirit. Instead of seeing them only in the guise of the person we think they have become, dig deeper. Assume nothing. For if an orange were only judged by the leathery texture of its surface, we would never know the fiery succulence that lies inside waiting eagerly to quench our thirst with the citrusy tang of tropical sunsets.

INSIGHTS

- For the dementia patient, the positive impact of joyful experiences lingers after the experience has been forgotten.

- Search through your loved one's past for clues that might trigger beautiful memories, like dear Monsieur Proust and his *petit madeleines*.
- By visiting your loved one frequently, you could be positively affecting their moods and behaviors.
- Do not underestimate your loved one's power to experience and retain the affection that you share with them.
- Do not overlook any opportunity, no matter how small, to bring a bit of joy into the life of your loved one.
- Although the impact of all you do for your loved one may not be outwardly obvious, never stop trying to kindle those tiny sparks of joy that lay hidden deep within their heart.

9

NATURE

Come forth into the light of things,
Let Nature be your teacher.
She has a world of ready wealth,
Our minds and hearts to bless—
Spontaneous wisdom breathed by health,
Truth breathed by cheerfulness.
                    —William Wordsworth
                    "The Tables Turned"

Nature is my eternal certainty, a comforting friend who has traveled close beside me as I have made my way through the world. When I am lost, she offers me a safe harbor among the giant sentries that fill her forests. When I am sad she wears a dress of snow-white petals and green moss to make me laugh and smile. When I rejoice, her winds play jolly airs in celebration. Her gifts never fail to refresh and sustain me.

I grew up in the countryside among the green, rolling hills of southern Ohio. My home was surrounded by thick woods, clear brooks, and wild, purple possum grapes that my friends and I ate right off the vine. Nature was everywhere, a part of my daily existence, a goddess to be worshipped and revered. As I grew, so did my love for all that she created: fragrant earth packed with worms, storms that brought downpours in cats and dogs, fiddle ferns that coiled on the forest floor and played sweet melodies to birds and bees alike.

I find it hard to imagine a life without access to the magnificence of nature. In today's technological world, it is easy to forget that we are part of her extended family, a distant cousin to all of her creations. We forget that we are living beings who require sunshine and fresh air in order to thrive. We forget that we are part of the continuum that gazes down upon us in the night sky. We forget that we too are stardust.

For many years the scientific community has recognized the potential restorative power that nature can have in our lives. Evidence exists that our brain waves actually change when we are surrounded by vegetation and nature. Over thirty years ago scientist Roger S. Ulrich became the first scientist to utilize an electroencephalograph (EEG) to monitor the brain wave activity in adults as they viewed photos of nature and then photos of urban cityscapes.[1] Results indicated that when we view lush scenes of nature, we have higher alpha wave activity in our brains, which results in a relaxed state of being and lower anxiety levels. It is important to keep in mind that participants in these studies were only looking at photos. Just imagine the calming effects that transpire when we are physically present and witnessing nature firsthand.

This news was not too surprising, since mankind has recognized this truth for thousands of years. Since the earliest days in China, Persia, and Greece, we have understood that contact with nature reduces stress and promotes well-being.[2] I think that most of us know this intuitively. So why do our modern healthcare institutions neglect this ancient understanding when constructing facilities? Why is our fundamental need to commune with nature not considered when creating care plans for the sick, elderly, and cognitively impaired? I may not know the answers to these questions, but I do know that we cannot rely on a facility or institution to connect our loved ones to the healing power of nature.

Physical and spiritual renewal cannot occur when we are closed up in a building with little natural light or fresh air. No, we need opportunities to feel the softness of grass under our feet and to touch the smooth bark of a crepe myrtle. I pity the person who never feels the soft warmth of sunshine on their face or smells the bright green fragrance of spring. No amount of environmental air filters or aerosol sprays can replace the smell of trees swaying in the wind on a soft summer's afternoon.

As I have told you before, in my early days as a caregiver my main focus was to ensure that Nan's daily physical needs were being met and that her environment was safe and secure. I am certain that today most of your energy is being spent in the same way. However, as time went on and I came to know other patients and observe their behavior, I soon realized that these issues are just baseline concerns. Yes, they are paramount to the life of the patient, but they are just the beginning, the foundation which enables them to experience the fullness of life. I came to realize that Nan needed more than just food, water, sleep, and help with rudimentary hygiene. She needed to engage with elements that would make her life rich and meaningful.

No life is one dimensional. In order to be fulfilled and find happiness each of us must have a multitude of experiences that reinforce our well-being. We must feel alive and a part of the world around us. We must experience simple joys like crisp autumn days spent under bright blue skies. Nature has the power to infuse our lives with an innate sense of peace. And this does not change as we grow older or become impaired. Just because they have limitations does not mean that the positive influence of nature cannot bring incredible happiness into the lives of our loved ones. Nature can elevate them from a state of merely *existing* into the soaring heights of feeling completely *alive*.

When I speak of Nan's well-being I am not just referring to her physical health. I am painting well-being with the broadest possible brush to include human attributes that run much deeper. I want the splendor of nature to help minimize her anxiety, generate positive thoughts, and promote a general feeling of happiness and peace. I know that you want the same for your loved one. Trust your instincts. Be guided by the intrinsic principles you know to be true. The joys of nature should not be forgotten just because an individual has dementia. In fact I believe that dementia magnifies the need to make this primal connection and has the power to touch sufferers very deeply.

I have a dream, a dream of a nursing facility that incorporates exposure to nature into its care plans and physical building design. At my facility, nature's serenity is brought indoors through large windows and skylights. All residents would have easy access to an enormous healing garden filled with plants and running water. Rooms would have windows equipped with glass shelving for potted plants and flowers. Residents would make regularly scheduled outings to the countryside. During warm months, dining outdoors would be commonplace and would only cease when the chill of autumn filled the air.

Unfortunately, I have never seen a facility that even comes close to fulfilling my dream. Although Nan has always lived in the best places that we could find, at the end of the day they still looked and felt like institutions. They have had limited outdoor space and minimal activities scheduled outside. So the solution, like so many others in my caregiving experience, was simple. I had to roll up my sleeves and get busy creating activities that would connect Nan with the natural world.

The first thing that I decided was that we do not have to actually be *in* nature to enjoy its beauty. For many years, each week my husband would take his mother for a long car ride deep into the countryside, far from the city streets and traffic noise. Nan had a particularly jaunty hat that she saved just for these occasions. It was taupe with a wide, black, grosgrain band at the base of the crown. Every Sunday before he left, my husband called out, "I'm off to drive Miss Nan." This joke never got old, because we both knew what a backseat driver Nan could be and that she was only happy when she had verbal command of the steering wheel. Toward the end of each ride they always ended up on the banks of the James River, along the same shore that Captain John Smith navigated on his way to the Jamestown settlement. They spoke of him each week and tried to imagine how he must have felt to be so near the end of his journey. If the weather is particularly fine, I sometimes packed a picnic and tagged along. Together the three of us sat by this historic shore with our car windows rolled down and the sunroof wide open. And here we enjoyed our lunch as the water lapped against this colonial shore and geese circled overhead just before gliding down to land on the smooth, brackish water.

SPRING

As each season arrives there are new and exciting ways to connect your loved one to nature. Spring brings the gift of flowers. Anyone who knows me will attest to the fact that I get a bit excited when it comes to flowers. They lift me up and brighten my spirits. Their growth cycle is a metaphor for life, which I think is why I love oriental carpets. In the center there is typically one flower in full bloom that is turning to seed and by the time it works its way through the foliage and birds to the outer design edge, the seed is once again a flower. Incredible beauty arising from a seemingly tiny speck of dust is nature at her most sublime. And spring is the beginning of this wondrous cycle.

I cannot think of anyone who does not respond to the perfection of a simple blossom. I incorporate flowers into Nan's daily life by making sure that she always has a cheerful bouquet in her room. Consider doing the same for your loved. When a vase isn't handy, a mason jar will do and can look especially charming when filled with spring tulips and daffodils. There is no need to spend a great deal of money or purchase flowers from a fancy florist. Thankfully a wide range of flowers are available today at reasonable prices. A supermarket bunch will be just as appreciated as an expensive bouquet. Or better yet, share flowers that you picked from your own backyard.

As the old rhyme goes, spring also brings showers. On rainy days Nan and I sit at the large picture window in her facility and watch huge raindrops create great muddy puddles. We talk about how lucky we are to be inside where it is warm and dry. Nan does not mind the rain because like any good farm woman, she appreciates the importance of a good, soaking rain. After all, "It is good for the garden."

When the weather is fair and the ground is dry, nothing is more enjoyable than having a picnic outdoors. Spread a quilt on newly mown grass and remember to bring along a folding chair so that your loved one has a comfortable place to sit. Bask in the beauty of the day. Smell the new grass and listen to the sounds of the birds and the insects, or better yet, feel the caress of a resurrecting breeze.

SUMMER

Nan and I have shared some of our happiest moments together in my backyard on summer afternoons. While I kneel and pull marauding weeds that have invaded my beds, she oversees my work and busily chats about whatever pops into her mind. Usually her conversations are about the nearby flowers or the birds at the feeders. Her favorite is the yellow finch to whom she is incredibly loyal. She even loves them in the autumn after their feathers have molted into a drab, olive brown.

Sometimes she speaks of her past gardens and how she used to love to can vegetables. During these stories I always hand her a clump of dirt so she can crumble it between her fingers. It is my hope that for one brief instant the cool Virginia soil from my backyard is transformed into the fertile soil of a faraway Ohio farm.

I take time to show her the flowers that are just budding and are sure to be a riot of color during her next visit. I sit her in front of my massive hydrangea bushes so that she can feel their leathery leaves and touch the blooms that have grown as big as cats' heads. Afterward we sit in the shade of ancient white oaks that were mere saplings when our nation was young. Sometimes I lay in the hammock while she sits beside me. And sometimes we cool ourselves with paper fans while drinking iced lemonade poured from a cornflower blue pitcher covered with a cotton doily in order to keep out the flies.

She and I both love summer's produce and eat sweet, juicy peaches, watermelon, and sliced warm tomatoes right off the vine. We rub herbs between our fingers and smell the heady scent of lemon balm and mint. We put sprigs of rosemary in our hair. We adorn ourselves with necklaces and crowns made from clover blossoms, like the kind I used to make when I was young. And for one glorious afternoon we are crowned as midsummer's queens.

AUTUMN

The mellow days of autumn are a gentler time with sunshine and golden afternoons as precious as honey spread on fresh warm bread. Nan and I love gathering leaves and saving them in a basket that she can take indoors. We place them in her room to remind her of the beauty of the season and the day that we spent together.

Sometimes we just sit outside and drink in the exquisiteness of a fall day busy with nonstop excitement—the last hooded warbler swaying on a milkweed pod, a blanket of crows scavenging corn that the reaper left behind, V-shaped formations of geese gabbling in the sky, the song of the last whippoorwill saying goodbye.

On days when Nan does not want to go outside or is particularly anxious, we still take time to sit by a window and look out on the trees and the grass. We have learned to enjoy nature any way that we can and anywhere that we can find it.

Since Nan's birthday is in October we always plan a small celebration and, if we are lucky, we honor her special day in the warm sunshine of an Indian summer afternoon. We laugh, sing, and enjoy a cake large enough to be shared with her neighbors and the staff at her facility.

WINTER

A day does not have to be sunny and warm to be filled with delight and surprise. Even in the dead of winter, when drifts of snow cover the ground, Nan and I still enjoy the beauty of nature. Since we can't spend time outdoors, we sit at the window and admire the bare trees whose branches are covered with snow and dripping icicles as sleet beats hard against our windows. We watch the birds that visit the winter feeders and the sunshine reflecting off the icy top of snow banks. We drink sweet, hot chocolate and talk of winter things like sledding, snowmen, and cozy firesides.

We also spend the winter months dreaming of the promise of spring by forcing flower bulbs to bloom. I find that amaryllis and narcissus work the best. We place the bulbs shoulder to shoulder in shallow bowls and cover them with small stones. Next we add water and before long we have a lovely display. Sometimes if the blooms become top heavy, we use ribbon to tie them to branches that I have found in my yard. When they are done blooming, I take them home and transplant them into the beds in my garden. Tulips and hyacinths can also be forced to flower, but first they must be tricked into thinking that they have experienced an entire winter season. I do this by placing them in my garage refrigerator for about two months.

In the late winter months, my mailbox becomes inundated with glossy seed catalogs. Nothing cures the winter blues better than leafing through pages filled with heirloom vegetables and annual flowers. Together Nan and I sit and choose our favorite flowers and plan where we will plant them in just a few short months. Then three weeks before the final frost we begin our garden in small pots that I make from newspaper that we set on her windowsill. Winter is a time for enjoying nature's quiet beauty as it slumbers and to look toward the spring wonders that lie just around the corner.

For me experiencing nature has always had a feeling of familiarity, like finding my way home after a long journey. It is haunted by the ghosts of my childhood. No matter what my dilemma it reassures me that all will be well in the end. It renews me physically, emotionally, mentally, and spiritually. It urges me to look beyond myself and remember that I am but one small cog in a giant wheel. I find this thought comforting as I make my way in the world: this notion that the world will still be here long after I am gone. It gives me permission to lay down my load and sit for a while so I can rest my tired back against the mossy bark of a sheltering tree.

Our instinctive need to be outdoors is so powerful that there are times when Nan and I have trouble making our way outside. As we reach the door of her facility, other residents who realize where we are headed clamber around us asking if they can come along. Unfortunately, I am only permitted to escort Nan outdoors. It is heart wrenching to tell them *no*, because I know that they don't understand why they can't join us outside in the sunshine. Once we are outside, I try not to look back at their faces pressed against the glass in the door window. Who can blame them for wanting to go outdoors and breathe in fresh air? I certainly cannot.

From this day forward, make a commitment to reconnect your loved to the replenishing power of nature. Make this promise a gift that you share together. Take them outdoors and point out every living thing that surrounds them. See the squirrels playing tag at the base of a tree, the flowers ladened with fat bumblebees, and the butterflies as light as tissue paper.

Make nature part of your loved one's daily life. Help them feel a part of her great cycle by celebrating each season of the year. Reintroduce them to the wonders of the landscape they knew as a child. Let their hands touch stones, soil, and soft violet petals. Let their nostrils breathe in the soft fragrant breezes. Let their hearts be lifted by the song of a lark. Let their soul be touched by the promise of rainbows.

In Victorian times, lovers sent their intendeds a message of devotion in the form of floral nosegays. Each flower spoke a language of its own, representing a feeling or promise for the future. Today this simple gesture has moved beyond poetic dreams and, as any flower enthusiast knows, has become a vocabulary all its own.

Often when Nan and I see a flower we stop and I will try to recall its meaning. If I know we will be spending time in a garden or I am taking her a bouquet, I will tuck *The Language of Flowers*[3] into my pocket for easy reference. I say to Nan, "Oh yes, there is a pansy which means 'loving thoughts.' And just over there is some alyssum which means 'sweetness of soul.'"

If I could, dear Nan, for you who so loves flowers, I would gather you a bouquet spilling with all the blossoms of a lovely summer's afternoon: daisies for *loyalty*, white chrysanthemums for *truth*, hyacinths for *constancy*, crocuses for *cheerfulness*, lavender for *devotion*, and of course rosemary for *remembrance*. Oh yes, I almost forgot the most important flower of all, the small sweet blue faces of forget-me-nots.

INSIGHTS

- Compelling scientific evidence proves that nature has the power to restore and calm our minds.
- When the weather permits, take your loved one outdoors so that they can experience the pleasure of fresh air and sunshine.
- Even if the weather is cold and rainy, you can still enjoy nature by sitting at a window with your loved one. Discover the loveliness that is present even on a gloomy day.
- Celebrate all the wonders available during each of the four seasons.
- Always have a fresh bouquet of flowers in your loved one's room.
- Have lunch alfresco when the weather is fair and the conditions are right.
- Visit a farmer's market and bring your loved one ripe summer vegetables and fruits.
- Share memories of past seasons. Remind your loved one how they used to celebrate each quarter-turn around the sun.
- Take your loved one to a park or sit in your backyard so that they touch and smell flowers, leaves, and grass.
- Place a bird feeder outside your loved one's window so that they can experience nature when they are unable to go outdoors.
- Use a suction cup to place a humming bird feeder on their window so that they can watch these delicate beauties drink.
- Collect autumn leaves and place them in a basket in your loved one's room.
- In the winter months, experience a bit of happiness by forcing spring bulbs into bloom.

- Make the commitment to share the wonders of the natural world with your loved one.

10

THE FIVE SENSES

Too often we underestimate the power of a touch, a smile, a kind word, a listening ear, an honest compliment, or the smallest act of caring, all of which have the potential to turn a life around.

—Leo Buscaglia

Think back and try to remember the last time you saw a fiery sky at sunset, heard the sad coo of a distant mourning dove, smelled sweet honeysuckle entangled in an ancient hedgerow, tasted summer's ripeness in a warm tomato picked fresh from your garden, or gently touched the hand of someone you love. Senses that were formed when we were in the womb remain with us until our final moments. They add magnificence and meaning to our lives. They protect us, teach us, and keep us tethered to the physical world. If I wrote a list of all the great pleasures of my life and the magical inspirations that have kept my feet moving forward, every item would emanate from one of my five senses. Their influence is fundamental in helping us interpret every aspect of the world around us.

Joy is not dependent on memory. Joy springs from our inner spirit and is often ignited by the splendor of our five senses. Remembering this simple principle gives us the ability to infuse happiness into the life of the dementia patient. We should take advantage of every opportunity available to reintroduce them to the tactile intensity of their senses.

You may think that I am oversimplifying things, being trite in fact. But think about how you interact with the world around you—the tastes, smells, and sounds that you find deeply moving. Ask yourself what experiences bring you pleasure: a favorite song on the radio, a hot cup of tea, a friend's smile? As caregivers we must remember that dementia patients are no longer able to control their experiences or create their own happiness. They are prisoners to whatever is laid before them. They are at the mercy of people like you and me, loving caregivers, who strive to keep them based in reality. Imagine what it would feel like to live in a nursing facility where creating sensory joys is not a top priority. What would you do if you could no longer cook your favorite foods, purchase your favorite flowers, or tune in your favorite radio station? Don't let your loved one linger in the desolation of their disease. Help them to utilize all of their senses in order to experience every possible pleasure. Create sensory joys that will fill your loved one's life with delights like small sacred offerings.

HEARING

> Music is a moral law. It gives soul to the universe, wings to the mind, flight to the imagination, and charm and gaiety to life and to everything. It is the essence of order and lends to all that is good and just and beautiful.
>
> —Plato

For as long as I have known Nan, she has loved music. So I knew from the beginning that this would be common ground on which we could meet and enjoy our time together. But I never fully understood the impact that music can have on a dementia patient until I witnessed an incredible phenomenon while she was living in a unit for the memory impaired. What I saw astounded and amazed me. And when it happened over and over again, I was convinced that it was nothing short of a miracle.

Nan's neighbors on the unit consisted of individuals from a wide variety of backgrounds. All they really had in common was that each was suffering from dementia or Alzheimer's disease. And this is why the following story is so remarkable.

Whenever I came to visit, we always took the time to sit on her comfortable loungers and listen to music on her CD player. Typically we left her door open, so inevitably our music would drift out into the hallway. Soon after beginning the first track, a visitor or two would arrive at our door in order to listen to a Broadway melody or an old Baptist hymn. Some would close their eyes and smile. Others would sway gently to the rhythm. Others would just stare into oblivion as if entangled in the entrancing net of our music. There were days when as many as ten residents would find their way into Nan's room.

I was not amazed that they loved our music, but I found it staggering that our visitors represented all stages of dementia. It did not matter if they were newly diagnosed or staring blankly into space; they were drawn to our music. It was as if they were reacting instinctively. For me, this was proof that long after it appears like a dementia patient is nonresponsive to external stimulus, their senses are still alive and engaged. They still have that spark that seeks out loveliness.

Two particular pieces seemed to have their own special magic. When we played these our attendance grew exponentially. Both were by Johann Sebastian Bach. First was Glenn Gould playing the *French Suite No. 5 in G major, BWV 816, Gigue,* a lively and happy dance. The second was the *Partita No. 2 in C minor, BWV 826, Sarabande,* a slow and poignant, almost sad dance. When these pieces were played the patients gathered not just in the doorway, but came deep into the room as if trying to find the music. I don't know if they were attracted to Bach's trademark mathematical rhythm, or if they were drawn in by the sheer beauty of the melodies. Perhaps it was both. All I know is that when Nan and I would play our Bach, patients gathered around us like the multitude of notes written on a page of sheet music. Music was a touchstone that was able to connect these patients to the outside world.

There are countless ways to bring the miracle of music into the life of your loved one. Consider taking your loved one to a local concert or accompanying them to a musical performance within their facility. Scan your local television schedule for upcoming musical programs. They need not be high-brow. Nan loves reruns of The Lawrence Welk Show that air on our local PBS station. Libraries offer a wide range of symphonic and chamber music performances on DVD and CD. If you have access to the Internet, consider downloading a personalized Internet radio station from a free service like *Pandora*. CDs of ocean waves or birdsong are another wonderful source of listening pleasure. Or better yet, why not place a set of wind chimes near your loved one's window so they can hear the music of the wind?

Music has the ability to deeply touch us, regardless of our medical condition. Don't underestimate the power of beautiful sounds to bring us together. Be creative. For as we all know, "Music has charms to soothe the savage breast."[1]

TASTE

Food is our common ground, a universal experience.

—James Beard

Each summer when the rhubarb leaves had grown to about twelve inches across, Nan would harvest the pink, celery-like stalks and begin baking rhubarb pies. Most bakers use it as a tart additive to berry pies, mostly strawberry, but Nan would make a pie filled with just the tangy sweetness of rhubarb. I don't know how she managed it, but even without berries somehow it always ended up tasting like fresh strawberries. This was the way she liked it best. And while I sat in the kitchen of her farmhouse enjoying a slice of pie baked early that morning, she would tell me all her "rhubarb secrets." "Don't harvest any stalks in the first few years. Remember that the leaves are poisonous. Be sure and cut it gently. Don't be greedy and cut it down to the nub. Leave some goodness behind for the plant's roots."

Nan's kitchen was both her laboratory and her classroom. Whether she was canning beans, cutting fresh Silver Queen corn off the cob to be frozen, canning tomatoes, or making homemade sausage, she was first and foremost a teacher. Her passion was imparting her knowledge and love of homegrown foods to anyone willing to listen. Under a clock made from a black cast iron skillet sat a long ancient harvest table that she kept covered with a plastic floral tablecloth. This was her pulpit. It was from here that she gave her lectures, with her hands folded together in front of her to mark the solemnness of the occasion. And all the while, on the stove, soft, fresh butter sat next to a container filled with bacon drippings that she liked to use when she cooked "just to add a bit of flavor."

Not long after she moved into a nursing facility and I was visiting her for lunch, I asked her how her food tasted. By this time she was restricted to a pureed diet and I found it hard to believe that the colored goo on her plate could possibly taste anything like the food that it was meant to represent. And I was correct. Her reply was one single word, "Slop." Although this caused a flurry of giggles from those around her, it made my heart sink. But what did I expect? How could a woman who was used to eating food fresh from the garden or her own grocery store possibly enjoy institutional food? Since I could not personally cater each of her meals, I decided in that moment to begin supplementing her diet with some of her favorite foods. If the facility could puree canned beans and different precooked meats, why couldn't I puree fresh watermelon, peaches, and ripe summer berries?

This small act had a huge impact on Nan's daily happiness. This was at a time when all her daily pleasures could be counted on one hand. Thankfully, she was still able to delight in the taste of some of her favorite foods.

Now every Saturday morning when the season is right, I go to my local farmer's market and select anything that looks particularly fresh or tempting and hurry home to give it a whirl in my food processor. Sometimes to make it palatable, I may add a bit of liquid, such as broth or fruit juice. Over the years I have learned that just about anything can be pureed. I even add a bit of milk to peanut butter and whip it up as a special treat. Nan adores chocolate ice cream, so I buy a premium brand and take it at mealtime in a small thermos that I bought especially for this purpose. Pimento cheese is another of her favorites that can easily be made in the food processor. The possibilities are as limitless as your imagination, especially if your loved one is not on a restricted diet.

Think of all the foods that your loved one has enjoyed throughout their life. Did they love a certain marinara sauce with spaghetti? Or did they prefer a long-roasted osso buco? Remember that their taste buds are not only a wonderful source of pleasure, but the ticket that may transport them back to happier days. Give it a try. I think you'll be amazed by their delight.

SMELL

> Smell is a potent wizard that transports us across thousands of miles
> and all the years we have lived.
>
> —Helen Keller

On Nan's farm, not far from a stand of ancient apple trees was a twenty-acre fence row completely tangled with wild honeysuckle. As luck would have it, the two would blossom at the same time, creating an incredibly intoxicating aroma that can only be described as sensual. To this day when I smell honeysuckle or apple blossoms, I am once again standing out by Nan's big garden with a warm, scented breeze blowing in my face and my feet resting on top of soft, damp clover.

I remember how Nan loved the smell of flowers, especially those that grew on her beloved farm. When she lived in a room of her own, I scented it with the smell of her garden—flower petals, earthy moss, and linens fresh from the clothesline. Now that she shares a room, I no longer do this in case the scent would be offensive to her roommate. So now my only choice is to scent Nan. All her soaps, lotions and shampoos smell like summer sunshine, or *Spring Rain.* I always make sure to spray her wrist with a very light body spray, so that she can easily touch it to her nose throughout the day. It makes her happy when people tell her how lovely she smells and she is always sure to comment on any fragrance that I am wearing. If I arrive for a visit and she seems impassive, I pull out my trusty bottle of Wild Honeysuckle and together we are transported to a patch of sweet earth just north of a field's edge, somewhere deep in the heart of Ohio's farmland.

SIGHT

> Never lose an opportunity of seeing anything beautiful, for beauty is
> God's handwriting, a wayside sacrament. Welcome it in every fair
> face, in every fair sky, in every fair flower, and thank God for it as a
> cup of blessing.
>
> —Ralph Waldo Emerson

My mother was an artist—a true sculpting, painting, "I'm off to my studio," artist. From my first days with her she taught me to look deeply at everything in my surroundings. I don't mean a quick glance to get a general view of things. No, my mother's ability to *see* things transcended the mere viewfinder through which most of us look at the world.

"What color is the barren brush along the back fence?" she would ask me. When I was young I simply would reply, "Brown." "Brown? No, look again," she would command as she squinted her eyes in the direction of the bushes. "See the grayish purple that highlights the woody stalks? The slightest hint of green left on last summer's growth? And the deep purple where the plant meets the earth? Look again." And so I would do just that. I would look again, closing both eyes into a mimicked squint. And suddenly I was really seeing, not a bleak brown bush filled with dead stalks and vines, but a plant that still held traces of a summer's wild celebration and the promise of spring's upcoming main event. As I grew older and understood the rules of this game, I went out of my way to try to see an obscure color that she may have missed, like that odd green in the sky just before sunset, or the hint of orange only visible when the sunlight shone through the blue vase that sat on her desk.

Today I have come to appreciate my wonderfully quirky, bohemian mother. Long after she has left my side, I enjoy lying in a hammock, staring up into the canopy of our old white oaks and counting all the incredible colors that I see. Her view of the world is now my second instinct.

So for me it seemed only natural to try to fill Nan's eyes with all the beauty and color that I could find. Because I was taught at such a young age to really *look* around me, this seemed only natural.

When Nan was still able to go out in public I would take her to art museums, borrow a wheelchair, and roll her through all the galleries. We took time to stop and examine each painting. Although she loved the soft colors of the impressionist painters, she was particularly drawn to the vibrant colors found in modern paintings and sculptures. I remember that we would sit for a very long time in front of anything created by Frank Stella or Mark Rothko. Was it the color, the movement, or the artistic punch that they delivered? I do not know. But I found myself asking Nan the same questions that my mother asked me all those years ago. "What do you see in this painting? What colors do you see? How does it make you feel?"

As time progressed and Nan's disease worsened we were forced to give up our afternoons at the museum, so instead we utilized the only art gallery that we had at hand; the prints in the halls of her facility are now our own private exhibition. We stop and discuss each print and painting just as if we are viewing a precious masterpiece from a world-famous collection. My goal is to encourage her to use her eyes and really *see* the world around her.

I use everything I can to infuse her life with beautiful colors and images. We spend hours looking through magazines and art books. Instead of using plain white napkins at mealtime, I bring brightly colored ones by Caspari to add cheer and create a festive atmosphere. We have long conversations discussing a bouquet of flowers at the front desk of the facility, the happy fabric print on a caregiver's shirt, or the mossy roof on the house next door. I encourage her to look around and be aware of every visual miracle in her surroundings. The lessons learned at my mother's knee have not only made my life richer, but have motivated me to pass this wisdom along to Nan.

TOUCH

> Let us touch the dying, the poor, the lonely and the unwanted according to the graces we have received and let us not be ashamed or slow to do the humble work.
>
> —Mother Teresa

As I round the corner from the lobby, there is Nan sitting quietly at the nurse's station tucked up in a pale blue cardigan and wearing her favorite pink slippers. When our eyes lock she raises her arms high into the air in anticipation of our usual hello hug. Our movements are reactionary, a desire so instinctive that neither of us would ever consider saying hello in any other way. Reaching out to show comfort or affection requires no forethought, just a natural concern and love for another person. In fact, touching is so natural that I am certain that you are already using it to comfort and show affection to your loved one. This tactile nonverbal communication cuts through everything for that one moment in time. Consider utilizing touch in the following ways.

- *Light Body Massage*: Dementia sufferers and other patients living in nursing facilities often spend many hours each day sitting or reclining in the same position. This causes continual pressure on the same muscle groups in their back and shoulders. Nan finds a gentle massage on her shoulders, neck, and upper back to be soothing and relaxing.
- *Foot and Hand Massages*: I massage Nan's feet and hands with lavender body lotion. This is nurturing to the skin and very relaxing. The scent of lavender has the added bonus of reducing stress.
- *Holding Hands*: Take every available opportunity to hold hands with your loved one and to remind them of the affection that you feel for them. Holding hands also helps make them feel safe and secure.
- *Back Scratching*: There is nothing that Nan enjoys more than having her back scratched. Even though she can no longer carry on a normal conversation, Nan still manages to let her feeling be known when it comes to having her back scratched. She moves and exhales in loud sighs until I have scratched just the right spot.
- *Brushing Hair*: Nan loves to have her hair gently brushed. She finds this to be so soothing that she typically falls asleep after just a few short minutes.
- *Pet Therapy*: Many facilities encourage well-behaved pets to come for a visit to cheer their residents. Touching and petting a dog or cat can not only be soothing, but can also broaden and reinforce your loved one's ability to show affection.

I'd like you to take a moment and picture in your mind the hands of your mother and father. I have no doubt that you were able to do this quickly. Even though I lost my parents many years ago, I can still see the details of my parents' hands. Sometimes they are easier to recall than their faces. Though stilled by time, they are stored in my memory.

I have a friend who has a wall displaying photographs of the hands of people whom she has loved throughout her life. Some are old and gnarled, while others are so chubby and new that you wonder how their fingers could even bend. Oddly her wall of hands is more moving than any wall of faces could ever be.

Hands represent our lives and tell our stories. Some tell of tending cows and operating machine presses, while others tell tales of quiet afternoons sipping tea from dainty china cups. Look at your own hands. Now look at the hands of the one you are caring for. Now join them together. Let your mind capture this image and tuck it away in your heart so you can remember it long after their face has faded from view.

Sometimes when I am with Nan, I feel as if I am flying a kite. There she is whipping around at the mercy of any passing breeze. And here I am, feet firmly planted on the ground, holding fast to her string, refusing to let go, fighting hard for those brief moments when I am able to conquer the wind. Sometimes my fight is hopeless and she is too far afield to be guided. Oh, but there are other instances when I am able to reach her, when the taunt string in my hands becomes a tether between our two worlds. These are wonderful moments—moments when she transcends her disease and regains her humanity, moments when she is in touch with her five senses, moments that she and I create together.

INSIGHTS

- Remember to utilize your loved one's five senses to connect them to the world around them.
- Equip their room with a radio and CD player so that you can listen to their favorite music.
- Try playing selections from J. S. Bach's *Anna Magdalena's Notebook* and watch how your loved one reacts.
- If you play the piano or other musical instrument, consider performing for the residents in their facility.
- Encourage your loved one to sing songs. Oh, and don't forget to join in.
- Prepare your loved one's favorite dishes and invite their friends to share the meal.
- Serve your loved a large selection of fresh seasonal foods.
- Select light, fresh fragrances to scent your loved one's home.
- Purchase toiletries for your loved one that smell fresh and clean.
- Encourage your loved one to look around and really *see*. Share magazines and art books that you think they would enjoy.
- Point out the beauty that surrounds your loved one.
- Utilize the power of touch to sooth your loved one by gently massaging sore muscles and tenderly brushing their hair.

- Hold your loved one's hand whenever you can. In the end, this is a gift that you will have given to yourself.

11

MIND GAMES

The brain is like a muscle. When we think well, we feel good. Understanding is a kind of ecstasy.

—Carl Sagan
Broca's Brain: Reflections on the Romance of Science

By now you understand that the Moment by Moment technique challenges us to do big things in small increments of time. Individually, minutes may seem insignificant, but when added together they become powerful opportunities for monumental change and happiness. A packet of flower seeds may not seem like much when emptied into the palm of your hand, but when sowed and tended, these tiny spores have the potential to become fields of exquisite beauty. Although our progress at times is difficult to gauge, we must remain steadfast in our commitment to tend and nurture our loved one's small moments of awareness. We must have faith that when gathered together, these moments have the power to make all the difference in the world.

Dementia is a serious business—so serious in fact, that caregivers spend the majority of their time worrying about the disease and all its symptoms. In this situation we forget how important it is for patients to have fun and pursue outlets for creative expression. I am lucky because when I begin to take life too seriously, Nan always seems to get me back on track. When she catches me hovering over her and worrying about her temperature, a new medicine, or her recent blood sugar spike, she will say to me, "Stop fussing." Even with all of my experience in dealing with this crazy disease, I still need to be reminded to calm down and not transfer my worries onto her. When she commands me to relax, I know that it is time for me to step back, slow down, and maybe even schedule a bit of fun.

We have all heard the expression, "If you don't use it, you lose it," and I am convinced that the same applies to the mental capabilities of dementia patients. No one would argue that exercise is essential to our health and well-being. So why would our brains be any different? In order to keep our synapses connecting, we have to do a bit of brain calisthenics every now and then. I realize that dementia is a progressive physiological disease whose advance is out of our control, but what's the harm in doing a few mental jumping jacks from time to time? When planning activities for Nan I focus on two key elements: artistic expression and game-playing. Not only have they proven to be of equal importance, but they have also been a great source of fun.

Artistic expression in its many forms is a potent way for memory-impaired individuals to communicate their emotions. As their verbal skills wane, picking up a paintbrush can be an effective way for them to share their feelings. As bystanders, we receive the benefit of catching a glimpse into how they perceive the world. Their feelings are given a voice that has been silenced by their disease. Their inner thoughts are translated into broad strokes of color. After all, art is one of the oldest forms of self-expression. I have seen dementia sufferers who had never held a paintbrush in their hand create poignant and meaningful works of art. Family members are often mystified when they witness their loved one's artistic talent for the first time.

Whereas art is a vehicle for self-expression, playing games offers the patient opportunities to problem solve and preserve their interpersonal skills. It also builds confidence and is a wonderful source for positive affirmations. Game playing builds camaraderie, creates happy memories, induces laughter, and most importantly, is entertaining. Provided that you are selective and introduce challenges that are commensurate with your loved one's particular stage of dementia, games are an optimal vehicle for providing mental stimulation.[1] But do not choose games that are too advanced or complicated for their current mental capabilities, or they could become angry or frustrated.

Whether you are playing games or creating works of art, consider the following tips to ensure a positive and happy experience:

- Choose a time of day when your loved one is at their best and most alert. Don't try to play a game right before naptime or late in the day when they could be experiencing *Sundowners Syndrome*.
- Make sure that the lighting is adequate and bright.
- Make sure that your loved one is comfortable and is not hungry or thirsty.
- Involve them in decisions regarding games and activities. Let them choose what they would like to do so that they feel that they are a part of the process.
- Choose games that are variations of those they have enjoyed in the past.
- Find a quiet spot where they can concentrate and not be distracted. Eliminate as much surrounding stimulus as possible.
- Turn off the television. This is probably the best piece of advice anyone will ever give you. Television does not encourage critical thinking. Although there are times when television is a great source of entertainment, all too often the constant drone of talking voices and noise becomes the soundtrack of a patient's life. If you have ever visited a nursing facility and seen a room filled with individuals staring blankly at a large television set, you will understand my point. I am particularly amazed when I see family members indifferently watching television with their loved ones. Surely there are more productive ways to spend time together, like playing games or sitting in the sunshine.

Nan and I have enjoyed a variety of game-playing and art activities over the years. But there have been numerous occasions when I have had to rethink my strategy in order to accommodate her ever-worsening dementia. Initially we were able to play more complicated games with rules that needed to be followed. She used to love matching the characters in Old Maid. But as her dementia progressed she was no longer able to do this alone, so we play the same game in a simpler and less challenging way. Now I help her match her Old Maid pairs. Likewise, she used to enjoy painting large bright pictures that filled an entire sheet of paper. Today because she can no longer hold a pencil in her hand, we look at paintings in books and magazines.

Remember that the goal is that your loved one feels successful and experiences the confidence that is achieved by a job well done. We want them to feel victorious. When one activity becomes too difficult, stop and create a less challenging variation. Once again I must remind you to be flexible.

The suggestions that I list below are just that—suggestions. Some will be far too difficult for your loved one to enjoy. Others can be tweaked to accommodate their current cognitive abilities. Because the stages of dementia are so vast and the individual variables so complicated, I've listed a wide variety of mind exercises in the hope that one or two will be appropriate for your loved one.

BINGO

Studies reported in the *American Journal of Alzheimer's Disease and other Dementias* found that playing bingo provides mental stimulation that is therapeutic for people with cognitive disorders. What is amazing about this study is that participating patients performed at a higher level for some time after the game had ended. According to caregivers, patients remained alert and more aware of their surroundings hours after playing bingo. [2]

This is particularly encouraging news if your loved one lives in a nursing facility where bingo is a common afternoon activity. Before Nan moved into a memory unit, she lived in an assisted living facility where bingo was taken as seriously as a high-stakes craps game in Monte Carlo. Every afternoon just before two o'clock, the halls were filled with bingo junkies hurrying to get a prime seat up front by the ball cage. This always surprised me until I found out why. In this facility, bingo was played for money! I discovered this one afternoon when I was organizing Nan's drawers and I found a sock filled with quarters. When I asked her where she got the money, she told me it was her "stash" and that she had won it playing bingo. Talk about positive reinforcement!

Once it became difficult for Nan to keep pace with the bingo caller, I went with her and together we marked her card. We became quite the bingo team. It didn't matter to her whether I was helping her or not, she still loved collecting a quarter each time that I told her to shout, "Bingo!"

FLASH CARDS

Flash cards provide endless possibilities for fun and entertainment, and because you create your own deck they can be customized to reflect the personal interests of the patient. Use white index cards and a black magic marker so that they can be easily read, and let your imagination run wild. Here are ideas for possible card decks.

- Word Play—Words have always been Nan's forte. For as long as I have known her she has carried a pocket dictionary in her purse. As a matter of fact, her love of the written word gave me the idea of creating flash cards in the first place. She retained the ability to read aloud up until the later stages of her disease. Whether we were traveling in a car or walking down the hall in her facility, she would call out the words that appeared on every sign that we passed. I noticed how proud this made her, so I created a card deck listing some of her favorite things, for example, Family, Surprise, Birthday, Garden, Puppy, Cake, and Togetherness.

- Simple Math Equations—These cards can be used to stimulate your loved one's long-term memory. For example, we all know from memory that $2+3=5$, since we memorized these simple equations in school. However, if given the equation $2+3+5=10$, we are forced to problem solve and utilize reasoning techniques.[3] Both equations use cogent techniques for stimulating thought processes; however, once again you have to remain sensitive to your loved one's cognitive level. The latter equation may only be effective in the early stages of the disease. Make sure that the equations are commensurate with your loved one's level of understanding.

- Colors—Go to your local paint or hardware store and select a variety of large paint chips that can be glued to flash cards. You can also cut photos from magazines, or use paints or magic markers. It is fun to ask the patient what colors they see and to think of objects that are that color.

- Birds—If your loved one enjoys being outdoors, print common bird pictures from the Internet and adhere them to index cards. Some of Nan's favorites are red cardinals, common house wrens, eagles, seagulls, yellow finches, and bluebirds.

- Sports—Print photos pertaining to their favorite sports activities and see if they can recognize the elements of the game—for example, team logos, baseballs, basketballs, or footballs.
- Flowers—Create cards that display photos of flowers that we all know—for example, geraniums, daisies, pansies, Queen Anne's lace, and lilies.
- Animals—Adhere photos of different animals to a set of cards. They can be domestic pets or exotic safari animals.
- Family Members—Create a deck containing photos of different family members and ask your loved one to recall their names.

JIGSAW PUZZLES

Working on jigsaw puzzles is a wonderful mental exercise and is an activity that your loved one can enjoy alone or with others. Select a puzzle that has the appropriate size pieces for both their vision and their cognitive abilities. Choose a theme that you know they will enjoy. If they like jigsaws, consider setting up a table in their room especially for their puzzles. Or if they live in a facility, ask the administrator to designate one table in the activities room for piecing puzzles. This will encourage others to join in the fun and create an opportunity for them to socialize with other residents.

READING ALOUD

Few things are more soothing than having someone read to us. Select short stories, poems, essays, or newspaper articles that you think your loved one will enjoy. You can either read to them, or you can ask them to read to you. As Nan's disease progressed and she could no longer hold an entire story or article in her mind, I resorted to reading selections from our Happy List.

DOMINOES

The game of dominoes promotes brain activity by promoting our ability to apply spatial reasoning. It is also an exercise in problem solving. Once again, dominoes is a game that can be played alone or enjoyed with other players.

BOARD GAMES

Select board games that your loved one has played in the past. Being familiar with the rules and object of the game will make the experience less stressful. Don't choose games that are too long and cannot be played in one sitting. Monopoly is far too daunting, whereas checkers and Parcheesi are more appropriate.

EXERCISE

It is common knowledge that exercise is good for the brain. It gets our blood pumping and is a wonderful stress reducer. For Nan, exercise is also a form of play. Together we point our toes, lift our legs, and raise our arms in the air. When she was able, we would take slow walks to exercise her muscles and work off nervous energy that often prevented her from sleeping.

If your loved one lives in a facility, check the activities schedule for the day and time of their exercise classes. Most classes teach patients how to exercise from a sitting position through the use of resistance bands and simple limb movements. If your loved one is afraid or hesitant, consider going with them for the first few sessions until they become more comfortable.

Don't assume that your loved one will automatically be escorted to exercise sessions. If you can't join them, contact the staff and request that they are included in future classes. If applicable, ask that someone accompanies them to the activity.

COOKING

If you have access to a kitchen, help your loved one prepare some of their personal favorites. Ask them to teach you their cooking secrets and together create favorite dishes from their past. Be sure to have everything set up and prepped so that the process moves quickly. Do all the chopping in advance so that there is no need for them to use a knife. When you are finished, sit down and share your creation with friends. Food is always a wonderful way to fellowship with those you love.

If they are no longer able to cook, ask them to help you frost and decorate homemade cupcakes or sugar cookies. Encourage them to share their creations with their friends and care workers. This is a heartfelt way for them to be able to thank all those who help them each day.

CRAFTS

Crafting is a positive way for your loved one to unleash their creative spirit. It builds self-esteem and promotes a sense of achievement. Crafting offers as many creative possibilities as there are patients. Just remember to select projects that reinforce their talents and interests. Help them discover that it is still possible for them to express themselves artistically. Reassure them that they still possess the power to create something beautiful. Here are a few ideas to get you started:

- Help them create objects using craft modeling clay. There are two types of applicable clay available at craft stores. Polymer clays come in a wide variety of colors, but require baking in order for them to harden. While other clays remain soft so they can be used again and again. Check with your local craft store to find the clay that best suits your situation.
- Flower arranging is a beautiful activity for a quiet afternoon. You can use fresh flowers from your garden or silk flowers from the craft store. Be careful to do all the cutting for your loved one so that they do not injure themselves. Containers can be anything from mason jars to plastic containers. Just secure a foam oasis in the bottom of a vase and let their imagination run wild. If you want them to create small gifts for their family or friends, consider

using laundry detergent caps as vases. They make nice containers for sweet little bouquets.

- Instead of carving a jack-o-lantern at Halloween, let them paint a face on the pumpkin. If necessary, you can outline a face for them and let them color in the features with magic markers or paint.

- Rubber stamps can be used to create a variety of projects. Just about anything can be stamped—for example, craft picture frames, fabric for pillows or aprons, or papers to make greeting cards. Purchase a variety of stamps and colorful ink pads so your loved one has a variety of colors and shapes to choose from.

- Help them make a wreath for their door at home or in the nursing facility. Purchase a round Styrofoam form from your local craft store and help them cover it with flowers that are appropriate to the season. During the holidays you may want to consider using inexpensive tree ornaments or red and green gum drops adhered with toothpicks. In autumn you may want to cover a wreath with autumn leaves and pinecones.

- If your loved one enjoyed needlepoint in the past but can no longer work on small projects, purchase kits that consist of a large grid plastic mesh with a preprinted design. Provide them with a large gauge plastic needle and acrylic craft yarn to fill in their project.

- Create a family photo album or scrapbook. Print copies of family photos on your computer and help your loved one create a personal scrapbook. If you need ideas, visit the scrapbooking section of your local craft store.

PAINTING

Because I was raised by an artist, when I am creating activities for Nan my heart always travels back to painting. I agree with Henry Ward Beecher when he wrote, "Every artist dips his brush in his own soul, and paints his own nature into his pictures."[4] I encourage you to put a brush in the hand of your loved one and see where it takes them. Let them express their love of color and life. Let them show you what they see when they look out into the world. Who knows, you may gain insights far beyond anything you could have imagined.

I suggest using good quality watercolors and thick, heavy, art paper. If quality paper is too pricey, heavy card stock that you can buy in reams at an office supply store is a nice alternative. I have found that a No. 6 brush is easy to manipulate and works well for both large and small projects.

As your loved one's abilities fade, trace outlines of objects on heavy-duty art paper and let them paint within the lines, or consider switching from paint to water soluble markers. But most importantly, encourage them to keep creating.

RECITING

Ask your loved one to recite a favorite poem, quote, or prayer. Nan loved reciting *The Lord's Prayer*, which became both a cognitive exercise and a supplication. Even if they are only able to remember simple nursery rhymes, that is fine. The point is to stimulate their minds and engage them verbally.

Spending time with those we adore in an atmosphere of fun and pleasure cultivates feelings of love and belonging. I am convinced that mind games have helped Nan stave off and cope with the progression of her disease. It has also fostered her pride and given her a feeling of accomplishment. Playing games and creating art have encouraged her to interact with others socially and be less withdrawn. They have been vehicles for her to express her innermost feelings. And in complete honesty, I've enjoyed it, too. During that one short hour I would forget all my worries and concentrate on what is truly important—that Nan is here today, enjoying her life and experiencing happiness. And if she happens to shout "Bingo" and wins a few extra quarters for her sock drawer, that just makes it all the better.

INSIGHTS

• Adapt the *If you don't use it you lose it* approach to dementia care.

- Encourage your loved one to be artistic with paints and drawing paper. This activity is a wonderful way for them to express their feelings and emotions.
- Whether doing a creative activity or playing a game, choose a time of day when your loved one is at their cognitive best.
- Select games that are in alignment with their abilities and cognitive aptitude. Your goal is to offer them a positive experience and to build their confidence.
- When visiting your loved one, always choose to engage them in a mental activity rather than watching television.
- Accompany your loved one to scheduled game activities at their facility.
- Support your loved one's bingo habit. Let them experience bingo's positive therapeutic effect by encouraging them to play.
- Create flash cards to stimulate your loved one's long-term memory.
- Read aloud to your loved one, or ask them to read to you.
- Encourage your loved one to exercise, even if they are only capable of making minimal movements with their arms and legs.
- Adapt games and activities that align with your loved one's interests or previous occupation.
- Recite favorite poems or prayers with you loved one, remembering to ignore mistakes or lapses in their memory.

12

COMMUNICATION

In the land of Gibberish, the man who makes sense, the man who
speaks clearly, clearly speaks nonsense.

—Jarod Kintz

In 1999, the BBC reported an extraordinary story of a bottle that was
found in the River Thames by a local fisherman. It contained a letter
written in 1914 by Private Thomas Hughes, a World War I British
soldier, to his wife. He had sealed his note in a ginger ale bottle and
tossed it into the British Channel. Sadly, two days later he died while
fighting in France. Unfortunately, Mrs. Hughes had died in 1979, so
the note was delivered to her eighty-six-year-old daughter, who was
only one year old when her father died. His sweet love note had taken
eighty-five years to reach its destination.[1]

In many ways I can relate to the feelings that Private Hughes must
have had when he tipped his ale bottle into the channel, hoping beyond
hope that somehow his message would find its way to his beloved wife. I
too send messages to someone far away hoping they will be delivered.
But instead of paper, my messages are written in the spirit of optimism,
placed in a bottle called *faith*, and flung into the turbulent sea called
Dementia. Some messages make it through, while others get caught in
an undertow and become entangled within the depths of unyielding
confusion.

When we hear the word *communication* we are certain that we
understand its meaning and feel that no further explanation is
necessary. Surely we did not get to this point in our lives without under-

standing what it means to communicate with another human being. The concept is simple. I transfer information to you either verbally or in writing and voila, we have communicated.

We also think of communication as missives and commands that we transmit out into the world. All we have to do is hit the *send* button and we have communicated. How simple can it be? However, to define communication on these terms oversimplifies the delicate transaction that occurs when we share our ideas with others. Communication is not only the process of sending information, but it is also the process of understanding what is being communicated.

Communication is an art that consists of two equal parts, the sender and the receiver. In order for the sender to have effectively transferred his message, the receiver must understand the incoming information literally and emotionally. Just because I send you information does not guarantee that you have correctly interpreted either my message or my intent. Incorrect assumptions occur all the time in our daily lives without our even realizing it. This can destroy relationships, create misunderstandings, and even have an impact on our professional careers.

Ensuring that the information that you are relaying to another individual is being correctly interpreted can be a tricky business. After all, no two people think exactly alike. Each of us has different mental aptitudes and unique life experiences that create a bias as to how we interpret the world around us. We are all looking out through different lenses. Our individual point of view is just that—ours—and filters how we send and receive information. You and I don't see the world from the same vantage point; therefore, I could inadvertently offend you with my words, mannerisms, or even my tone of voice. If we are from different cultures, the likelihood of a misunderstanding rises even further, since phraseology and word meanings vary greatly across socioeconomic and cultural lines.

At this point you might be thinking, "This is all well and good, but what does this have to do with dementia?" Well, I'll tell you. Communicating with the dementia sufferer is the number one problem plaguing caregivers, and can be an unending source of frustration. Our inability to verbally connect with them often blocks any attempt that we make to enhance their lives. I am confident that you are spending a great deal of energy trying to close the communication gap that exists between you and your loved one. For me this has been one of the greatest challenges that I have faced while caring for Nan. I work hard each day coaxing her to perform even the simplest physical task, like opening her mouth so that I can position her dentures. You can talk to a dementia sufferer until you are blue in the face, but if you don't approach them correctly or they are having a bad day, there is nothing that you can do to cut through the haze. Concentration cannot be forced on another individual and the more you try, the less likely you are to succeed. I know this is true because I have the mental scars to prove it.

Of course, no one has all the answers, but there are ways to communicate that will at least stack the deck in your favor. These techniques were born from trial and error, watching the professionals and applying a strong dose of good old-fashioned common sense. It is my hope that by using these tools I will be able to help you communicate more effectively with your loved one.

Ordinarily, if you and I are having a conversation, I can determine if you understand my message by watching your body language and listening to your verbal responses. We don't even give it a thought. It is instinctive. But when we attempt to communicate with an individual who is memory impaired, it is difficult to ascertain what gets through, let alone if they understand our meaning. Sometimes when I tell Nan something, I get an appropriate response. But there are other times when all I receive is a blank, vacant stare, while other times she meets me somewhere in the middle by responding, but not to the question that I asked her.

I have no way of predicting which will happen. It feels like a coin toss. So even if your loved one nods in agreement, don't assume that they understand what you are trying to tell them. And don't think that just because you repeated your message ten times, they have correctly interpreted your meaning. The communication model for information sharing with a dementia sufferer has little in common with how we transfer information in our normal daily life. To think otherwise would be a mistake.

Dementia tips the balance of the communication equation, requiring us to be responsible for both the sending and receiving of information. This necessitates extra thought on our part because this is not our natural way of communicating. Normally, we say our piece, pause, listen, and wait for our turn to speak again. But when dealing with a dementia patient you often have to deliver your message in nontraditional ways. It requires that you act mindfully and take the focus off yourself and devote all of your attention to the receiver, to your loved one. You must constantly rethink your communication tactics in order to maximize the likelihood that you will be heard and understood.

Not long after Nan began having cognitive issues, I asked her neurologist if he knew what it felt like to live inside Nan's head. I asked him to what extent she had control over her thoughts and actions. He told me that most of the time her thoughts whirled around in her mind as if they were in a blender. I try to remember this when I am attempting to tell her something important. His explanation necessitates my empathy and understanding. It begs me to be patient. This insight has become my secret weapon when trying to penetrate the ether of Nan's consciousness.

Think about the most recent exchanges that you have had with your loved one. Were they effective? Were you tempted to raise your voice? Were you so frustrated that you wanted to just throw up your arms and walk away? In the end did they understand what you were trying to convey? Or were you both exasperated at the end of your encounter? If your answers make you cringe, don't be too hard on yourself. All caregivers struggle in the area of communication because there is no formula or *right* way to ensure success, but I encourage you to consider the following advice.

COMMUNICATION ADVICE

- Speak in short clear sentences. Don't overwhelm the patient with lengthy explanations and reasoning. Leave out the *why* of what you are hoping to accomplish. Remember, their ability to reason has been curtailed and additional information will only result in additional confusion. For example, there are times when I simply say to Nan, "Let's eat."
- When you ask your loved one to do a physical task, break the request down into small easy-to-follow steps. Don't just say, "Get out of bed." Instead gently guide them through the process. First tell them to "Sit up"; then "Put your feet on the floor"; then "Hold onto your walker"; and then "Stand up slowly."

- If they become frustrated or agitated when you are trying to convey information, stop and walk away. Do not argue with your loved one. Leave them alone for five or ten minutes so that they can calm down and relax. Most likely by the time you return they will be in a better and more cooperative frame of mind.

- When having a conversation with your loved one sit face-to-face. I have found that Nan and I are much more likely to connect if we are sitting close to each other and watching each other's faces. Sometimes we sit so close to each other that our knees almost touch. This enables our eyes to meet and for her to focus on my moving lips. Eye contact always helps create a connection between two individuals.

- Speak in words and phrases that they used prior to their dementia. For example, when Nan was displeased with something she used to express her disdain by using the adjective *ridiculous*. So now when she refuses to let me put her dentures in her mouth, I quietly tell her that if she goes all day with no teeth she will look *ridiculous*. More often than not, this does the trick.

- Don't ever assume that they have correctly interpreted what you are trying to tell them. If they are able, retest their understanding by asking them to repeat information back to you. Remember you are responsible for both sides of the communication equation.

- Schedule video phone calls with family and friends who live far away. This is not only helpful for the patient, but it can also be a relief to those who do not have the opportunity to visit frequently.

- Maintain proper hydration levels. Hydration is a key factor facilitating cognitive clarity and awareness. When Nan is dehydrated, she becomes confused, anxious, and defiantly noncommunicative.

- Monitor your loved one closely for possible infections. Because their systems are so sensitive, even a small infection can have an enormous impact on their daily life. Take their temperature regularly and if they begin to show signs of a fever, contact their physician immediately. Nan is particularly vulnerable to infections and can display drastic behavioral changes with even the slightest rise in her temperature. Sudden changes in your loved one's demeanor can signal an infection.

- Don't plan visits or activities late in the day if you think that your loved one suffers from Sundowner's Syndrome.

If you are caring for someone with dementia, I am certain that you have heard of Sundowner's Syndrome. Almost every individual whom I have met who has dementia suffers from some form of this syndrome. In Nan's case, this was one of her first symptoms to appear. In the late afternoon and early evening she became increasingly angry, noncooperative, and aggressive. Although she exhibited mild variations of these behaviors throughout the day, they escalated as evening approached.

Over the years I have heard many different explanations as to why this occurs. Some professionals attribute this change to the reduction of natural light. Others think that a contributing factor is the end-of-day frustrations of care workers. I am not a scientist but having witnessed countless Sundowner's episodes in a wide variety of people, I think that it all comes down to changes within their brains in relation to their internal clocks. Around the time that Nan began to experience Sundowner's her sleeping patterns changed drastically and she began to confuse her days and nights. Although there is no real cure, research has shown that increasing a patient's exposure to light may diminish the symptoms.[2]

As Nan's dementia progressed, her Sundowner's symptoms tapered off. This was a relief because for a short time it was necessary to manage her behavior with the use of a mild sedative so that she would not harm herself or others. I strongly recommend that you speak with your physician if you believe that your loved one is experiencing symptoms of Sundowner's Syndrome.

- Monitor medication changes. If you notice an abrupt change in your loved one's ability to communicate or assimilate data, investigate what medications they are taking. Make sure that they are receiving the proper dosages. Make sure that a change has not been made without your permission. Many times throughout Nan's illness it has been necessary to actually reduce her dosages or omit a medication altogether. Be sure to speak to your physician anytime that you witness abrupt changes in your loved one's personality, sleep habits, or communication skills.

- Maintain healthy blood sugar levels. Here is yet another factor that can affect your loved one's ability to communicate and enjoy their life. Dementia sufferers are extremely sensitive to high and low blood sugar levels that can directly impact their confusion and anxiety levels.

- Be flexible. As you know all too well, dementia patients have good days and bad days. Don't try to convey important information on a day when they are overly tired or are having difficulty with their normal routine. Also, choose a time of day that they are typically the most alert and mentally active.
- Keep a positive attitude. Remember that the patient is an emotional sponge and is affected by both your verbal and nonverbal cues.
- At mealtime encourage your loved one to sit at a table and eat with family members or other residents. Don't relegate them to the sidelines by having them eat alone in their room or in front of the television. Mealtime is a wonderful opportunity for them to communicate and engage in social interactions. Eating with others also brings a sense of belonging into your loved one's life. Do everything in your power to create a warm, beautiful, and loving meal setting. Make mealtime an event that they look forward to. I think that if you take my advice you will also see an increase in their appetite.
- Stay calm and relaxed. If you feel yourself becoming stressed, walk away. Don't overreact to anything that they say or do. Do everything in your power to remain serene. You are more likely to gain their cooperation if you maintain a gentle, quiet demeanor.
- Change your tactics if necessary. If you find that you are not connecting, try a new strategy. If you are still unsuccessful, take time to pause and begin again tomorrow.
- Never stop trying. This is my most important piece of advice. No matter how bad things get, keep trying to find new ways to break through their shell. Experience has taught me that they are still trying desperately to remain connected to you. Do everything in your power to help make this happen. Never stop trying to help them remain in the world around them.

I don't want to lead you to believe that every time that Nan and I sit together we always have a meaningful and purpose-filled conversation. Our reality is quite the contrary. In the early days it was comparatively easy to make a connection. By using a simple commonsense approach I was somewhat successful gaining her cooperation and relaying important information. However, as time went on it became increasingly difficult to get my point across. Unfortunately, I had to lower my expectations.

Today by using the methods I have mentioned, I usually am able to make her understand what I am trying to communicate. I pay close attention to her body language and nonverbal clues for confirmation that we understand one another. I also gauge my success by the tone of her voice when she is talking in "Nan Speak."

Nan Speak is a term that my husband and I coined to describe the language that Nan has come to utilize when verbally communicating. It isn't really English, although there may be a few familiar words in the mix. No, to be honest it is a language of gibberish. Nan has always been a great talker, a communicator extraordinaire, and this personality trait did not diminish when she began suffering from dementia. She still loves to talk, but now she speaks in a new language of her own creation. What began as a few odd nonsense words is now a full-blown language complete with verbal inflections and heartfelt explanations. To someone who didn't know her, it would sound like the babble of a baby. But to me, someone who interacts with her every day, it is a rich language that expresses her moods and inner feelings. I truly think that she believes that she is speaking in English. I can tell when she is happy, sad, angry, or despondent. So I make every effort to respond appropriately by either offering my concurrence or my comfort.

I particularly love it when she uses *Nan Speak* to tell me something that tickles her fancy or she finds particularly funny. These are my favorite interactions, because right in the middle of her story she will stop and laugh uncontrollably. Then once she is able to catch her breath, she picks up right where she left off and finishes her monologue. Usually she tells me about something that she witnessed during her usual daily routine. I know this because if I ask her if it happened that day, she nods and throws her head back in uncontrollable laughter.

When I am listening to Nan tell me stories in her private language, I become the receiver of all that she has to share. It feels like I have been let in on a grand secret or have gained membership into an exclusive club. It reinforces what I know in my heart—that like the rest of us, she just wants to be heard. We all want to tell the stories of our daily lives, so I sit and listen attentively until she has finished her recitation, after which she settles down; then it is my turn to speak of happy things and my news for the day.

Not everything she tells me in her *Nan Speak* is positive and happy. Sometimes she is sad and her eyes fill with tears. When this happens I sit patiently and let her finish. I tell her that I completely understand and then slowly begin to steer the conversation onto lighter topics. I might say, "Yes, but you're too smart to let that bother you. And after all it takes all kinds to make a world." Or I might say, "Weren't you lucky? You did the right thing and everything worked out perfectly." Usually responses like these will change the tone of the conversation and get her back on a more positive track. Granted, this was more difficult when she was first diagnosed and she was constantly repeating her concerns. In those days everything she said reminded me of a needle that was stuck in the groove of a record. My point is that no matter what their stage or circumstance, we should always try to lift our loved ones up by taking gentle control of the conversation. We should try to tenderly guide their thoughts onto cheerful topics.

Nan is also the master of nonverbal communication, a maestro in fact. Without uttering a single word she has the ability to make her moods and feelings known through her actions and body language. For example, one day when I arrived for a visit, I found Nan sitting quietly with one of her favorite dollies in her lap. I asked her how her day was going. Her answer was strong and clear. While looking me square in the eye, she picked up her doll by the foot, slowly stretched her arm out over the side of her Geri-Chair and promptly dropped her doll head first onto the floor. No Nobel Laureate in Literature could have expressed their feelings more clearly or succinctly. I got the message.

Not every nonverbal clue that we are given is as blatant as the incident with the doll. Most are more subtle and may show in our loved one's facial expressions, body posture, or eye contact. You are the best one to assess the nonverbal clues of your loved one. You understand their idiosyncrasies and natural behaviors. Be a detective who is on the lookout for any signs that might reveal how they are feeling. If they rub their head, ask if they have a headache. If they keep lifting their legs up and down, ask if they have a leg cramp. If they keep squirming around, ask if their back hurts. I have found that when it comes to pain Nan has the ability to answer my inquiries, even if it is just with a nod or shake of her head. Remember, each of their nonverbal actions is worth investigating.

I hope that by now you are realizing that the Moment by Moment technique applies to every aspect in your caregiving experience. It can be utilized to bring joy, create emotional memories, drink in the beauty of nature, and yes, even help you communicate effectively with your loved one. Remember to think in terms of short snippets of awareness and time. Break every request into small uncomplicated steps. Avoid long explanations and minute details. Remember, you cannot win a debate or obtain buy-in from a dementia patient. Instead, speak simply and clearly. Refuse to be baited into an argument. Fight the natural urge to explain the *why* to everything that you are trying to communicate. And always, always remember to be patient and kind.

INSIGHTS

- When communicating with a dementia patient we are responsible for both sides of the communication equation—that is, the sending and receiving of information.
- Pay close attention to your loved one's verbal inflections and nonverbal responses when you are conveying information.
- Remember to speak clearly and in brief sentences when speaking to your loved one.
- Remember to break down commands into small, easy-to-follow steps.
- If your loved one becomes agitated or upset, walk away and try to communicate later.
- Sit face-to-face when speaking with your loved one so that you can make eye contact.
- Assume nothing. Check repeatedly to ensure that they understand the information that you are trying to communicate.
- Don't plan visits during the later part of the day if they suffer from Sundowner's Syndrome.
- Remember to be flexible. If one communication tactic is not working, try another.
- Remain calm and positive. Remember your loved one is able to sense your frustration and impatience.
- If your loved becomes upset by a certain topic of conversation, gently steer the discussion onto lighter subjects.

- Leave out the *why* when conveying a message to your loved one.
- If your loved one creates their own language for communicating, embrace it by listening closely to every word that they say.

13

DIGNITY

Every life deserves a certain amount of dignity, no matter how poor or damaged the shell that carries it.

—Rick Bragg
All Over but the Shoutin'

Dementia is a world of disappearing things. Over time your loved one's memories are tossed one by one into a turbulent sea. The first to go are the words to a poem that they learned in grade school, lines that were once so familiar that it seemed they were chiseled in stone. Next to go are the dates that stack as high as the clouds—saints' days, holidays, anniversaries, and birthdays. Then come their yesterdays, last weeks, and the proper place for objects. Faces come next, those in old photographs and those they see every day. Until finally, when there is nothing left to offer Poseidon, their dignity is heaved overboard never to resurface again.

Dignity is an intrinsic trait defined by self-respect and humanity, a noun that states the common link between all men. Dignity is not earned, but instead it is an entitlement given to us at birth, a tie that joins us to the rest of humanity. Dignity is our right to be heard, understood, and treated fairly. It defines each of us as beyond value and worthy of all that is excellent. Whether or not we choose to honor its existence in another person is for each of us to decide. But no matter what actions we take, we cannot rob another individual of their inherent prerogative to possess it. Respect must be earned, while dignity is our birthright. Just think of the power that would be unleashed if each of us would venerate the dignity possessed by everyone we meet. And I believe that this gift, given to us on the day we were born, is ours to keep for all the days of our lives.

In modern Western society we want to live long but we don't want to grow old, which is an oxymoron if ever I've heard one. We enthusiastically worship the goddess of youth and underestimate the wisdom and talents of our elders. The marketing term *antiaging* makes me cringe each time I hear it. It sounds more like negative propaganda than a promise to smooth away facial wrinkles. When I hear it, my heart cries out, "There is no shame in growing old!"

I prefer to remember the painter Manet, who while on his deathbed, painted the flowers that his friends brought him. They are gentle works, radiating his eternal optimism and joy. And there is Grandma Moses who did not pick up a paintbrush until she was seventy-eight or the writer Harriet Doer who published her first book at the age of seventy-three. To them I cry, "Comrade!"

Is it any wonder that these accomplishments and others like them are rarely praised in a society whose great marketing machine continually pumps out campaigns glorifying youth? How can this constant barrage of slogans and celebrity worship not brainwash us and affect our attitudes toward the elderly? Lately it seems like the only time we hear much about senior citizens is when commentators are discussing the escalating costs of social security in relation to the burden it places on the government's budget. The time that I have spent in nursing homes and the battles that I have fought on Nan's behalf have solidified my opinion that we need to reexamine how we view the elderly in our society. They deserve to be treated with the dignity earned from a lifetime of contributions and sacrifice. After all, each of us should be so lucky as to live well into our golden years.

We need to be made aware that not every culture in the world agrees with our view of the elderly. Not every country relegates old people to the outer boundaries of society. For example, Japan honors its elderly with a national holiday. *Respect for the Aged Day* is celebrated each year on the third Sunday in September. In India elders within a family are respected for the sacrifices that they made on behalf of the next generation, so young people seek their good wishes, *Sankalpa*, and blessings, *Aashirvaada*. Why, even the ancient Greeks considered the care of the elderly as a sacred duty to be carried out by grateful children.[1]

If you will remember, dignity was a key component in my mission statement. My primary goal in all I do for Nan is to maintain her health and dignity. I want her to feel that she is still valued and plays an important part in the lives of those whom she loves. She deserves this. Throughout her life she fought hard to preserve her dignity. She experienced hardship and neglect. Often she had no one who was willing to be her safety net. She has been frightened, disappointed, and experienced injustice. But the persona Nan showed the world revealed nothing of these trials. All the wrongs and adversities that she suffered became mere footnotes relegated to the bottom of the page, written in tiny print almost too small to read. Nan was a woman of divine character and dignity. She gave respect in abundance, and now it is time for her to be repaid in kind.

The Parable of the Good Samaritan from the Bible says,

> A man going down from Jerusalem to Jericho was attached by robbers. They stripped him of his clothes, beat him and went away, leaving him half dead. A Samaritan, as he traveled, came to where the man was; and when he saw him, he took pity on him. He went to him and bandaged his wounds, pouring on oil and wine. Then he put the man on his own donkey, brought him to an inn and took care of him. The next day he took out two denarii and gave them to the innkeeper. "Look after him," he said, "and when I return, I will reimburse you for any extra expense you may have."[2]

Typically when we think of this story, the golden rule comes to mine. "Do unto others as you would have them do unto you." And yes, this is true. But there is another layer to this parable, one that for me transcends the obvious. For I believe that the Samaritan returned the wounded man's dignity. His personal character compelled him to be kind to the injured stranger, and by providing a place for him to rest and heal, The Good Samaritan gave the traveler back his self-respect. What was stolen by the robbers was returned by the Good Samaritan. When we offer our empathy and kindness to a loved one with dementia, we ourselves are acting like the Good Samaritan by protecting and restoring their lost dignity.

Imagine if you were no longer able to dress or feed yourself, remember the date, or administer your own medicines. What if there were times when you didn't even know where you were? Now imagine that you required assistance for all of your daily ablutions, from bathing yourself to choosing what clothes you will wear. What if you relied on others to schedule your appointments and even decide when you needed a haircut? I know I would find this dehumanizing, degrading, and frankly, embarrassing. I would feel helpless and at the mercy of everyone around me. It would be almost impossible for me to see myself or my situation in a dignified light.

I have an old photograph of Nan that I have always loved. She is about eighteen years old and has her thick blonde hair pulled back in waves behind her ears. She is sitting on the top step of an old-fashioned porch next to a bush heavy with verbena blossoms. Nan is wearing a delicate white blouse and soft-colored skirt and is smiling into the camera. Her demeanor is not pretentious or haughty, but her dignity is palpable. I keep this photo in a silver frame atop a stack of my favorite books and look at it often to remember Nan's innate poise and elegance. Little did she know all those years ago when she was posing for this photo, that she was setting the tone for her later days. She was making an unwritten codicil to her will, telling her daughter-in-law, who wasn't born at the time, exactly how she wanted to be treated during her final days.

This photo exemplifies how I want the world to see Nan, composed and poised. Even though she may act a bit silly at times, I don't want her physical appearance to look out of control. I want her to look neat and tidy. I want her to be seen in the best possible light at all times. This is especially important, since care workers never knew her when her mind was sharp and her body was healthy. They only know her as she presents herself today.

Of course it is impossible to keep Nan perfectly groomed every minute of every day, but I make sure that she always looks her best. She looks clean and fresh, her hair is brushed and her clothes are laundered and wrinkle free. I am dedicated to my mission statement and determined to honor the young woman who sits inside that silver frame in my library.

ADVICE FOR MAINTAINING A DEMENTIA PATIENT'S DIGNITY

Bathing

In a Facility:

- Although Nan's facility provides soap and other hygiene products, I buy Nan freshly scented, extra-moisturizing body washes.
- I provide Nan with a rich skin moisturizer, gentle deodorant, and cornstarch-based baby power so that her skin is hydrated and smells fresh.
- Communicate your hygiene concerns to the aides who attend your loved one. Nan has a plastic-handled caddy that holds all of her bathing and grooming products. This makes it easy for her helpers to transport her personal products to the shower room. You might want to include a laminated checklist inside the caddy detailing your particular concerns.
- Nan's face tends to be dry and flakey, so I provide a rich facial moisturizer that is applied in the morning and at bedtime.

At Home:

- Safety should always be the first concern when bathing an individual with dementia.
- Install a shower wand and shower chair in their bathroom so that they can sit while bathing.
- Never allow them to bathe unattended. As an additional precaution, turn down the temperature on your hot water tank so that they are not inadvertently scalded.
- Create a bathing schedule. Depending on their continence issues, twice a week should be adequate.
- Use multiple washcloths. Use a new cloth for each section of their body.
- Make sure that the shower floor is not slippery. This includes the area outside the shower.
- Install appropriate shower bars or handles so they can move around easily and safely.

Hair

- Choose a style that is short and simple. Complicated hairstyles have a tendency to appear untidy. Styles that require heavy doses of hair spray can look messy after they have been slept on. Also, if the patient perspires, their hair can get gummy, tangled, and appear unkempt. Likewise, if the style is complicated, they will typically have to have their hair shampooed or *done* once a week. This is an impossibly long time to keep an ornate style looking fresh when you spend a great deal of time resting your head against a chair or a pillow. From my experience, before the week is out, elaborate hairdos tend to look like fright wigs.
- Gentlemen's hair should be cropped short for comfort and ease.
- Stop the chemical treatments. I can't tell you how many residents in both Nan's assisted living facility and nursing home receive permanent waves and hair color treatments. Usually this is because the family wants their loved one to maintain their old hairstyle and look as they did in the past. Remember that our goal is to ensure that they are neat and clean, not glamorous. Why subject them to the chemicals and the time it takes to apply these solutions to their hair? Embrace the natural color and texture of their hair. There are endless short hairstyles to choose from. Nan's hair is cut into a short bob and, honestly, it has never looked better.
- Having a simple, well-cut style makes it possible for your loved one to have their hair washed when they are in the shower. This is critical in order to avoid cradle cap and other chronic scalp conditions. This is especially important during the summer months when they are more likely to perspire.
- Since I can never be certain of Nan's mood on the days she is scheduled for a shower, I provide her helpers with a shampoo and conditioner combination. This ensures that her hair is cleaned and conditioned in one easy step. Because Nan has an especially dry scalp, occasionally I ask the aides to massage her head with a deep penetrating hair conditioner.
- Don't use blow dryers, curling irons, or other heated appliances when styling your loved one's hair. Their movements are often unpredictable, which could cause either of you to be burned.

Shaving

- With today's grooming products, it is easier than ever to keep both men and women's faces free of unwanted hair. For men, purchase a rechargeable electric razor so that it is not necessary to use a razor blade on their face. For women, purchase a small, personal, battery-operated razor for the removal of any unwanted facial hairs.

Clothing

- Make sure that your loved one gets completely dressed every day. Their morning routine should be to rise, get dressed, and have breakfast. Don't let them linger in their bed clothing like an individual who is sick or has no purpose in life.
- Their wardrobe should be functional. Select clothing that can be easily removed and is comfortable for them to sit in for long periods of time. Although discount stores offer a large array of inexpensive garments, I have found that when I purchase moderately priced clothing they hold their shape and last longer, which in the end saves money.
- Purchase trousers one size larger than they would typically wear. Since Nan wears adult diapers, this makes it easier to dress her.
- Purchase clothing that is machine washable, wrinkle resistant, and seasonally appropriate.
- When you are changing out their wardrobe at the start of a new season, pass a discerning eye over their clothing. Eliminate all items that no longer look fresh and tidy. When items become stained or worn, eliminate them from your loved one's wardrobe.
- Keep clothing mended and in good repair.
- No matter the season, have sweaters on hand for them to wear. Elderly people tend to become cold easily.
- Reconsider your loved one's undergarments. In order to keep Nan comfortable, I eliminated her bras and replaced them with white cotton camisoles. Not only does this keep her warm in the cool months, but it also wicks perspiration away from her skin when she becomes hot. Select undergarments that are roomy and made of 100% cotton.

- Have multiple robes handy for them to wear before and after bathing. Light terry cloth robes work well for men, while women can wear housecoats that snap down the front. Remember we want the robes to be easily slipped on or removed.
- Night attire should be soft, comfortable, and loose at the neck. Remember that your loved one lacks the ability to solve problems, so if they become entangled in their nightclothes, they may have difficulty freeing themselves. Never buy them anything that is tight at the neck or wrists.
- If your loved one is bedridden, consider this: For women, purchase nightgowns that are soft and pretty. Then cut them down the back from the neck to the bottom hem and create your own personal hospital gown. Machine surge or hemstitch the long, raw edges so that the fabric does not fray. Sew a soft ribbon on either side of the back neck opening so that it can be tied loosely. Men's nightshirts can be altered in the same fashion.
- Over the years I have learned that appropriate socks are important for maintaining good foot health. Nan is diabetic, so I take what she wears on her feet very seriously. I select white, cotton knee-highs that are not too tight. I choose white because they can be bleached and kept impeccably clean, while knee-highs serve as a barrier to help protect Nan's shinbones. Since she is no longer able to walk, the muscles in her legs have atrophied to the point that her shinbones are prominent and exposed. Longer socks serve as an extra layer of protection against bumps or scrapes when she is being transferred.
- If your loved one lives in a facility you must decide who will do their laundry—you or the facility. Granted it is more convenient for the facility to do their laundry, but consider this: Most facilities comingle all the residents' clothing. They wash clothes in hot water using harsh detergents and they certainly do not use fabric softeners. In their defense, this ensures that germs are eliminated. However, industrial laundering reduces the life of each garment and increases the likelihood that your loved one's items will be misplaced or lost. Consider doing their laundry yourself. By using mild detergents and fabric softeners, their clothing will feel better next to their skin. I have a dedicated suitcase with rollers that I use for the sole purpose of gathering and returning Nan's clothing.

Footwear

- Your loved one should always have either slippers or lightweight shoes on their feet. This is essential for their warmth and protection. Even if they are no longer able to walk, you still must protect their toes and feet from injury. I have seen many patients who have had their toes broken in wheelchair accidents or while they were being moved or transported. Even though Nan is confined to a Geri-Chair, she always wears a pair of substantial slippers.

Eyeglasses

- If your loved one wears glasses, designate a specific place for them to be kept after they have been removed. Provide a case marked with your loved one's name so that they do not become scratched or damaged. Strive to keep them in good repair. I say strive because I know from experience that this is no easy task. Nan's bifocals are constantly out of alignment. In order for her to see clearly out of her bifocals, they must sit properly on her face. I found myself spending so much time rushing out to have them readjusted that I purchased a second pair for her. Now I rotate them so that she always has a pair in optimal condition.

Tooth and Denture Care

- Maintaining proper oral health for a dementia patient is a tricky business. Most likely they are unable to endure lengthy dental appointments, which increases the likelihood that they will develop tooth decay or other oral health problems. It also becomes difficult to persuade them to brush their teeth twice a day. This is an area in which many caregivers give up. Many patients that I encounter have breath smelling of tooth decay and gum disease. Today there are toothpastes available that can be swallowed. So if you are having difficulty getting them to brush their teeth and rinse their mouth, this is an option that you might want to consider.
- Most dentists will provide mouth checks for patients who are unable to tolerate an entire dental exam. Remember to do this whether your

loved one has their own teeth or wears dentures. Check with your regular dentist to see if this service is available.

- If your loved one wears dentures, remember to help them brush their gums daily with a soft toothbrush made specifically for gums. Once again, if necessary use toothpaste that can be swallowed. Also, be sure to use denture-cleaning tablets that kill germs and have the highest whitening power.

- Make sure that your loved one's dentures fit properly in their mouth. Ill-fitting dentures can cause gum and mouth pain. As we lose weight, our gums also shrink in size. So make sure that your loved one's dentures are still comfortable for them to wear. If they become too large, consider having a liner made so that they fit more comfortably. Proper-fitting dentures are also less likely to be removed and accidently lost. I always place a small amount of adhesive on Nan's dentures to ensure a secure fit.

- My goal is to have Nan wear her dentures every day without fail. First, I want her to remain accustomed to the feel of having teeth in her mouth. She began wearing dentures long before she was diagnosed with dementia, so she is used to wearing dentures. But I realize that at some point in the future I may not be able to convince her to wear her dentures. I want to push that day as far into the future as possible. Second, I think that it helps her to maintain her dignity and positively impacts the image that she projects into the world. Nan just doesn't look like herself without her teeth. Third, her speech is clearer when she is wearing her teeth. And fourth, wearing teeth aids in chewing and food digestion.

Fingernail and Toenail Care

- It is imperative that you keep a dementia patient's fingernails trimmed and filed. This will prevent possible injury to themselves and to others. Often they will lash out at aides who are trying to help them. By keeping your loved one's fingernails trimmed you are decreasing the likelihood that care workers will be scratched.

- I suggest that you put all your loved one's foot-care needs into the hands of a nurse or a podiatrist. Most facilities have a podiatrist who makes regular visits. Have a standing appointment every four to six weeks to have their toenails trimmed and their feet thoroughly examined. This is especially important if your loved one is a diabetic or has circulatory problems.

When I was young, each morning before my father left for the office, he would stop by the kitchen table where I was finishing my bowl of cereal and say, "Today at school, act like you are *somebody*." I have never forgotten his call to dignity. I have never forgotten his gentle reassurance. And so each time I lean over to kiss Nan before I leave I whisper in her ear, "Remember that you are *somebody*." When I say these words I feel my father smiling behind me, proud that his sense of honor is being passed on to this small, helpless woman. And this is how it works. Dignity alive in one is passed to another, and then to another, and so on down the line, until it is repeated so often that it becomes a part of who we are and how we view our place in the world.

INSIGHTS

- Strive each day to maintain the dignity that befits your loved one's lifetime contributions.
- Because dementia causes erratic and often silly behaviors, make every effort to ensure that your loved one does not look foolish or wild.
- Encourage your loved one to act like *somebody*.
- Pay particular attention to their hygiene and grooming habits. Make sure that they bath frequently, have their hair cut at regular intervals, and are clean-shaven.
- Purchase clothing that is comfortable, attractive, and machine washable. You want your loved one to be easily dressed and undressed.
- Whenever possible, choose garments that are made of 100% cotton.
- Make sure that your loved one's feet are always protected by slippers or lightweight shoes.
- Keep their eyeglasses in good repair so that your loved one's vision is clear.
- Encourage them to wear their dentures every day.
- Have their feet examined regularly by a podiatrist.
- Accord your loved one the same dignity that you would wish to receive if you were in their situation.

14

SPIRIT

I find letters from God, dropped in the street, and every one is
    signed by God's name,
And I leave them where they are, for I know that wheresoe'er I go,
Others will punctually come for ever and ever.

                    —Walt Whitman
                    "Song of Myself"

The older I get the less I feel restrained to think of spirit within the confines of a specific religion or dogma. Instead, I see the grace of God, or a Higher Power, in the heart of many denominations and faiths. Whether we seek spirit outside of ourselves or from within, the desire to uncover the meaning of life lives within each of us. This intangible and mystical force is inside you and it is inside me. It is the essence that joins us to the continuum of the universe. It is the force that elevates everyday existence to higher levels of consciousness. Spirit is infinite and ever present, the path through which we relate to all of humanity and make the most of our time on earth.

Spirit travels to us through the mystery of grace. Grace is the sweet breath of God that swirls all around each of us. It touches everything in our lives. Grace is the love and goodness that exist in all of life's situations. It is the pathway to inner peace and immeasurable gratitude. Even if we do not acknowledge it, grace is always present. It is ours to call upon or to set aside. It has been with us every moment since the day we were born. The face of grace looks like wisdom, forgiveness, kindness, and compassion. It wraps its arms around us and always lifts us up. It cannot be scientifically counted or measured. It is as ethereal and as intangible as mist. Grace is that whisper of awareness and truth that humbly connects us to all living things. It is omnipresent. Even when we turn our back and crouch in the darkest corner, grace is there, patiently waiting to lead us back into the folds of eternal love. Just because we pay it no heed does not mean that it is absent. After all, the stars that we cannot see in the brilliant light of day are still burning as brightly as they do in the blackness of night.

For years I asked myself the question that has plagued believers down through the millennia, "How could God have allowed this to happen?" Born from anger and resentment, it sat in the back of my mind only to rise to the surface whenever I was tired or upset. How could God in all his wisdom bring such suffering onto one of His flock? Nan's faith was strong, as was mine; it seemed like God had forsaken us. I felt we were alone in a small boat in the middle of a thick fog. Then on one seemingly ordinary day a sweet kindness answered my question forever.

Nan had developed a large goiter on her thyroid and the doctor had ordered an ultrasound in order to check for further abnormalities. This was scheduled as an outpatient procedure in a large medical facility adjacent to our local hospital. At this point, although Nan was still able to transfer from her wheelchair into the front seat of my car, she often refused to stand up once she was in a seated position. Because she was not accustomed to being in the outside world, she easily became distracted or afraid. When planning doctor's appointments, I always had to add additional minutes to our travel time, just in case I had trouble gaining her cooperation.

On this particular day Nan broke her all-time record for stubbornness. It took twenty minutes for me to convince her to move from the front seat of my car into her awaiting wheelchair. I was just about ready to throw in the towel, when she finally relented and stood up. Along the outside of the facility there were benches for people who were waiting to be picked up from their appointments. I didn't know it at the time, but a woman on the bench was closely watching our exchange. As I wheeled Nan into the facility, I didn't even notice her. Little did I know it then, but I was passing by an angel.

The scan went beautifully, but I was dreading what lay ahead. Now I had to work a reverse miracle and try to coax Nan back into the car.

After about three unsuccessful attempts, I heard a soft gentle voice behind me say, "I saw that you were having trouble before, so I went inside and bought her a little present in the gift shop. Maybe it will grab her attention so that she will listen to you." I turned to see a small wrinkled woman with a broad smile and kind eyes. There in her outstretched hand was a doll wearing a crocheted dress and matching hat ornamented with a dangling price tag reminiscent of Minnie Pearl. I almost cried.

This perfect stranger was empathetic to both my frustration and Nan's medical condition. She had taken it upon herself to try to help. And now for the best part, it worked! Before long I had Nan safely settled in the front seat holding onto her present. I offered to pay the woman for the doll, but she would not hear of it. She was just glad to be of help. I was limp with gratitude.

Although this occurred many years ago, I have thought of this exchange countless times since. A woman whose name I don't even know saw that Nan and I needed help, and with no benefit to herself, came to our rescue. She made me realize that God is caring for Nan through all the special people that touch her life. Nan is a catalyst that brings out the very best in others. Now I vigilantly search for these angels. And to my wonder I have come to realize that Nan is the daily recipient of an endless stream of Godlike behavior, beginning with her caregivers and professional medical team, stretching all the way down to a kind, unknown woman sitting on a bench outside a busy medical facility on a warm summer's day.

Glimpses of grace are all around us every day of our lives. But if we are to experience its wonder, we must change our focus. We must become attuned to the joy that grace can bring into our lives. We must break down the barriers of our heart and become open to the possibilities of unlimited gratitude and love. We must shift our attention from the measurable tenets of the material world and take notice of the often-overlooked mercies that lay in our path. Like the morning you felt that your friend was in pain and after telephoning, you learned that she was in need of help. Or the day you took the long way home from a college class and met your future husband. Or the afternoon a kind stranger gave a doll to a woman and her daughter-in-law in a doctor's office parking lot. Or when you found a pressed flower tucked between the pages of a poetry book that your late mother used to keep on her nightstand. But remember to tread lightly. Sometimes grace arrives in packages so small that you almost let them pass by, like puddles after a thunderstorm, the song of the skylark, or the smile on the face of a friend.

> Amazing Grace, how sweet the sound,
> That saved a wretch like me!
> I once was lost but now am found,
> Was blind, but now I see![1]

At times we are called upon to become the grace makers. We are asked to listen to our inner voice and become the ewer by which others receive and experience God's love. Caregiving is like that; born from a heart filled with empathy and compassion, you allow the healing powers of the universe to work through your spirit. The help you give your loved one is an outward demonstration of grace and all her mysteries. You become her hands because she has none. You become her voice because she has none. You are both the receiver of her gifts and the conduit by which she is passed onto others. By making your life part of this continual circle of giving and receiving, of appreciation and sacrifice, you open your heart to acts of love that will come back to you tenfold.

I realize that not every life is guided by the principles of spirit and faith. Many wonderful individuals use science alone to define their time on earth. When I speak of the spiritual needs of a suffering individual, I am defining *spirit* in the widest possible terms, and not specifically to any religious affiliations. I am referring to the part of us that questions life's meaning. I am referring to our essence and our innate need to find comfort and peace. To neglect this aspect of the human experience just because the patient does not worship a traditional god would be short-sighted. We are greater than our living cells. And when we fall ill, we try to fit our new experience into a construct of life we understand regardless of our beliefs. This common link is our humanness and the consciousness that all of mankind shares. Each of us, no matter our beliefs, seeks love, acceptance, community, and happiness. When we are sick, even though our physical body is attacked, our inner core still laughs, cries, grieves, and hungers to be fed spiritually and emotionally.

The grace that surrounds Nan is so obvious that at times I can almost hear it humming. It is conveyed through a gentle touch, an efficient nurse, or the face of a visiting child. Nan is known for her love of children. When families bring their little ones to visit, they always make a special point to spend time with Miss Nan. Watching Nan laugh and jabber with the children brings joy to everyone watching. Her happiness becomes our happiness, spreading as if by magic. It seems like ever since Nan's world has been reduced to small moments, she has gained the ability to appreciate every little grace surrounding her. It is as if she is living from blessing to blessing, and in these small moments when I am with her, I catch small glimpses of heaven on earth.

When caring for someone with a chronic illness, it is much easier to attend to their immediate physical concerns rather than the needs of their spirit. After all, the first rule of triage is to stabilize the body. Consequently, their spiritual needs are often overlooked and pushed to the wayside. But in reality, these two needs overlap.

It is reasonable to assume that when someone is diagnosed with a serious illness their entire belief system is rattled with the impact of a seismic earthquake. Finding spiritual meaning among the rubble is difficult—especially when battling physical challenges. This makes it easy for you to lose your way and think that God has forsaken your loved one and you. I think that this is why the road to acceptance is often so wrought with pain.

The essence of everything I do for Nan is an attempt to reach her on a spiritual level. Yes, I attend to her physical concerns, but in reality that is a very small part of what I do for her. As I have discussed in previous chapters, I want her to remain part of the world around her and retain a sense of life's precious meaning for as long as possible. I want her to feel that she is still vital and has much left to contribute. I want her to experience joy, feast with her five senses, and see the majesty and grace alive in nature. I want to help make up for the links that have fallen from the chain that connects her to all that is peaceful and beautiful. I want to create emotional memories that will fill her heart and offer her a sense of peace.

One of my favorite writings on spirit is from a story called "The Great Spirit" written by Native American Zitkala-Sa:

> When the spirit swells my breast I love to roam leisurely among the green hills; or sometimes, sitting on the brink of the murmuring Missouri, I marvel at the great blue overhead. With half-closed eyes I watch the huge cloud shadows in their noiseless play upon the high bluffs opposite me, while into my ear ripple the sweet, soft cadences

of the river's song. . . . My heart and I lie small upon the earth like a
grain of throbbing sand. Drifting clouds and tinkling waters, together
with the warmth of a genial summer day, bespeak with eloquence
the loving Mystery round about us. . . . Here, in a fleeting quiet, I am
awakened by the fluttering robe of the Great Spirit. To my innermost
consciousness the phenomenal universe is a royal mantle, vibrating
with His divine breath. Caught in its flowing fringes are the spangles
and oscillating brilliants of sun, moon, and stars.[2]

I suggest that we make it our goal to remember to minister to the
entire person. Let us strive to help their whole being deal with their
limitations. Let us do everything in our power to support them both
physically and emotionally, so that they may calm the struggles that they
may be facing. We are not comprised of two separate compartments,
one physical and the other spiritual. No, they are entwined and tangled,
creating our unique personality and perspective of the world. One part
cannot be ravaged without the other being affected. They are much like
two hands folded together in prayer, interlocking fingers that work together for absolution.

Our belief system is radically challenged when we are struck down
with an illness or are facing death. Throughout her entire life my mother was a devout Christian. I never saw her waver regarding her beliefs.
After she died, her doctor spoke to me about the last conversation that
they had before she passed away. She asked him if he thought God
existed and if there really was life beyond this physical plane. Thankfully the doctor assured her that, yes, he felt that there was a God, and
explained that during his many years practicing medicine he had witnessed profound events that supported the possibility of an afterlife. He
said that she visibly calmed after hearing his answers. I have thought of
this conversation many times over the past fourteen years. My mother
showed me what it feels like to be dying. She taught me that fear can
sneak into your heart regardless of your religious convictions.

Sometimes when I am sitting with Nan, I think of my mother's
questions. And without being asked, I give Nan the affirmations that my
mother longed to hear. I try to offer her spiritual comfort and remind
her of her connection to all that is good and kind. I remind her that God
has not forgotten her and that he has sent us a splendid day as proof of
his love for her. We hold hands and I say prayers for people and things
that I know mean a great deal to her. Since she can no longer relay her

thoughts, I focus on what I know to be the truths of her heart. We give thanks and pray for her family and children, the well-being of others, and the many glories that surround us at that moment. And then of course we listen to her beloved hymns, her *prayers* as she used to call them. These devotions sung in a small room in a nursing home in Virginia could not be more meaningful if they were heralded in the largest cathedral in Christendom. Grace is all around us all of the time, just waiting to nourish our hungry spirits.

In order to be able to touch and feed the inner spirit of your loved one, you have to honor the fundamental tenets of their belief system. Don't assume that their lack of outward understanding means that they no longer feel and respond with a depth of spirit. Fill their lives with the ceremonies and traditions that they have practiced for a lifetime. Remember that religious traditions link us to our pasts, offer comfort, and tether us to concepts larger than ourselves. Read to them from the Bible or recite prayers of mediation. Honor Catholic saints' days and the holy Feast of Easter. Celebrate the Jewish New Year, Rosh Hashanah, by giving thanks for the past year and praying for the year to come. Provide the food and prayers for Shabbat dinner on the Jewish Sabbath. Read aloud the seven Unitarian Universalist Principles. Or commune as Zitkala-Sa did with the miraculous pulse of the Great Spirit. But most importantly, do everything in your power to provide your loved one with the answers to my mother's questions.

Many times just before rounding the corner to enter Nan's room, I have overheard a loving conversation she is having with a care worker. Sometimes they are singing, other times just humming, but more often than not they are praying. I always stop so I don't interrupt their unplanned worship. When she moved in I hung a small wooden cross above Nan's bed so that when she enters her room she will be reminded of Christ's love for her. But I also did it for this very reason: so that Nan would never miss an opportunity to be reminded of her faith by those who enter her room. Hopefully, when seeing the cross, a visitor will recognize that Nan is a believer and join her in fellowship, much like the sweet workers whose prayers surprise me when I make an unplanned visit. Surround your loved ones with clues to their faith, like a rosary, a Yakama, or a small wooden cross—not just for them, but also for others to see.

My time with Nan has become a series of grace-filled experiences. Although I know in my heart that I have brought joy into her life, I sometimes feel that I am the true benefactor of our time together. By listening to my heart and striving to give her wonderful moments, I too have had the pleasure of experiencing the simple joys of being alive. I've become filled with enthusiasm for small, uncomplicated gestures and view each new experience in a more positive light. As I searched for entries for our Happy List, I could not help but be grateful for every entry that I wrote. I was reminded that a life well lived need not be complicated. Whether collecting autumn leaves or eating fresh strawberries, Nan and I connected to the world around us and grew closer to each other. I see Nan as a shining catalyst for grace going forth into the world. Being with her during her darkest hours has allowed me to develop an inner strength and through grace to connect with God.

As the days go by, my life is becoming more and more interwoven with Nan's. I see that we are separate threads weaving the same cloth, weft and warp. Back and forth the shuttle passes. First to come is a thread of *joy*; next a thread of *love* passes through the heddle. Back and forth the shuttle passes. Our days are woven into tapestries of tender mercies and quiet exhalations, cloaking us in love. Two separate lives tightly joined on the eternal loom of grace.

INSIGHTS

- Recognize that when someone is ill or cognitively impaired, they still feel the need to connect with the world on a deep and meaningful level.
- Pay attention and search for the Godlike behavior that surrounds your loved one.
- Place visible signs of their spiritual beliefs in their surroundings so that visitors can join them in fellowship.
- Celebrate the rituals of your loved one's religion or beliefs.
- Do not neglect the spiritual needs of your loved one in lieu of daily chores and checklists.
- Remember to nourish your own spiritual needs while caring for your loved one.

- Know that God has not forsaken you or your loved one, but continues to guide and protect you during these trying times.

15

EMOTIONAL SECURITY

Could a greater miracle take place than for us to look through each other's eyes for an instant?

—Henry David Thoreau
The Complete Works of Henry David Thoreau

The emotional brain responds to an event more quickly than the thinking brain.

—Daniel Goleman

When caring for a dementia patient, your life becomes a series of imaginings. I imagine lost days, now so long ago, spent at the old farm. I imagine summer afternoons when we sat under the big, golden, maple tree between the big barn and the old tool shed watching white sheets and odd socks flapping on a taunt clothesline. I imagine the sound of your feet as they tread across the creaky, wood floor leading from the front parlor into the dining room. I imagine the sound of the old screen door slamming shut behind me, a welcoming sound that told you that I had arrived. I imagine your old tabby cats, Granny and Tom, circling around my ankles as I stepped off the worn stone threshold into the big white barn. I imagine the wet tangy smell of moss and fermented apples that filled my nostrils as I climbed down the steps into your root cellar. I imagine the look on your face the day that you understood that you were slipping away. And now I try to imagine what it feels like to be you and to no longer be able to remember your dear farm, or even recognize yourself in a faded Polaroid photograph.

I wish I could emotionally transport Nan back to the old place, the place where she felt emotionally safe and secure. I want her to be surrounded by its beauty and feel that certain calm that can only be experienced in the tranquility of the quiet countryside. I want her to gain strength from all that she has accomplished throughout her life and all the people whom she has loved and have loved her in return. I want all that has preceded this moment to gird her against her current challenges. I want her to feel the restorative peace that she experienced while walking down the lane on the edge of the west field, breathing in the scent of cornstalks growing under the sheltering, Midwest sky.

I realize that this is an extremely lofty, if not impossible goal. How do I give someone with this incredibly difficult disease a feeling of comfort and safety? I know that offering her any kind of emotional security is nothing short of a herculean task. Although I may not be able to hand it to her in a tidy package, I can try to shape her environment in a way that will allow feelings of safety and security to flourish. But like so many other elements that embody dementia, this goal is ethereal and at times can make me feel like I am trying to lasso mist.

When I speak of emotional security in relation to dementia, I am referring to a relaxed sense of safety that allows the patient to openly experience the joys that surround them. By creating an emotionally secure environment, you are unlocking the door that imprisons your loved one. You are pushing aside worries and fears, freeing them to experience more positive feelings. It is a vital step in the process of achieving your mission statement.

In Nan's case there has proven to be a direct link between her happiness and her sense of stability and emotional safety. And this makes sense. After all, how can she experience joy if she does not feel safe in her surroundings? How can she recognize and respond to beauty if she is worried or afraid? How can she begin to communicate her feelings if she does not trust the people around her? How can she be in touch with her inner spirit if she feels vulnerable?

Creating a safety net for an individual who does not outwardly communicate or relate to the world around them is incredibly challenging. Of course the main difficulty we face is our loved ones' lack of short-term memory. All our efforts and achievements are often lost in the blink of an eye. Consequently, we have to offer reassurance and love over and over again. We have to be consistent and vigilant. We have to keep filling their bucket despite the gaping hole in the bottom.

I continually strive to make every detail in Nan's life act as a counterbalance to her disease. I try to offset each negative and horrific attribute of dementia with a positive action. I try to create a calm retreat where she can find shelter in the middle of a whirling storm. It is a task that is never complete, a project that never ends. Each day I work to offer reassurance in an attempt to offset her confusion and despair. When she feels confused I want her to feel soothed. When she is afraid I want her to feel comforted and reassured. And for each remaining day of her life, I will be there piling my efforts, one on top of the other, hoping that in the end I will have made a difference.

I may not have the power to wave a magic wand and make all of Nan's fears and worries evaporate, but I can make her world conducive to internal calm and peace, much like providing water and sun to a growing plant. By paying close attention to her reactions and controlling several important variables, I at least offer her a chance of happiness.

I never know for certain what Nan is thinking, so I have to watch her reactions and listen closely to any information that she is able to convey. Like everything else in the swirling cauldron of dementia, it was easier to inculcate emotional security in the early stages of her illness when she was better equipped to react to physical and emotional stimuli. But even now, years later, I still work to insulate her from the trauma of fear and confusion by closely monitoring several key aspects of her life.

CREATING EMOTIONAL SECURITY

- Keep the patient's environment neat and orderly and create a daily routine for the patient that is based on their natural rhythms and inclinations.

  In order for any of us to feel secure, we must have some semblance of order and routine in our lives. This is especially vital for the dementia sufferer. When your head is swimming with mad thoughts, your world already feels chaotic. You certainly don't need anything else adding to your confusion. Set a daily routine and stick to it. Ensure that their mealtimes, bedtimes, and wake-up times are the same each day. The patterns you create by developing a workable daily timetable will create a calm and predictable environment that will foster and nourish you loved one's overall sense of security.

- Provide your loved one with a security object that they can carry with them.

Soon after moving into her first facility Nan became fascinated with the dolls belonging to other residents. She saw them being cuddled and carried around throughout the day. She loved looking at all the "babies" and sometimes she would even try to snatch them from their owner's arms. This caused such a ruckus that I think it is best to leave the details to your imagination. Let's just say that eventually we had no choice but to buy Nan her own dolly. Buying a child's toy for his bright and intelligent mother was a turning point for my husband. He could no longer deny the reality of her situation. She had entered into her second childhood. To his credit it didn't take long for him to come around once he witnessed the comfort his mother received from her "baby." Since then, her first "baby" has acquired quite a few siblings and now Nan holds her family of "kids" in a daily rotation, even while she is sleeping. Over the years she has also been given quite a few stuffed animals. Her current favorite is a stuffed horse named Rainbow Chaser.

- Ensure that everyone on your loved one's care team is competent and kind.

Remember that everyone who comes in contact with your loved one has the potential to impact their sense of security. If you employ aides to help tend to their needs, interview them carefully to ensure they are not only qualified for the position, but also interact with your loved one in a positive, loving manner. Everyone who steps into life should project a kind and tender energy. Efficiency is wonderful, but it is not the only qualification to look for when selecting a care worker. Check their references and have them spend monitored time with your loved one before making a final decision. Watch how well they relate to one another. Regardless of the candidates' credentials, trust your instincts.

- Act as your loved one's voice.

Nan constantly struggles to express her emotions and feelings. To get her point across she uses whatever method is available to her. She may shout. She may cry or she may rely on a litany of nonverbal cues, like raising her fist or rolling her eyes. Each one of these actions is her way of attempting to be heard and understood. It is my responsibility to stay alert, not take anything personally, and recognize that her feelings are valid. I always try to get to the bottom of whatever seems to be bothering her and assure her that I will resolve the situation. I tell her that I will be her voice and act as her advocate.

Not long ago Nan's shin had become scraped on the top of her bone. It looked as if her legs had been dragged across the bottom edge of a table while she was reclined in her Geri-Chair. When I asked the nursing staff how this happened, they said that they were unsure, since no worker had come forward to report the incident. Later that afternoon Nan and I were sitting outside during the aides' shift change. As a particular girl passed by, Nan lifted her injured leg in the air. I asked her if this girl knew how she hurt her leg. As I spoke she kept moving her leg up and down. When we were back indoors and I was getting ready to leave, Nan and I approached the aide and politely asked if she knew how Nan's leg had become scraped. The aide looked flabbergasted and explained to me that it was an accident and that she was so sorry that Nan had been injured. She also apologized directly to Nan.

This incident showed Nan that I was listening and that I had heard her. She saw that I had taken the necessary action to protect her and that she could count on me to make things right. Thankfully, we have experienced very few instances like this one, but I still pay close attention to all of Nan's responses, no matter how small or seemingly unimportant.

- Constantly remind the dementia patient of how much they are loved.

The best and most important way to instill emotional security in anyone we love is to give of ourselves and spend quality time with them. You know this from raising your family. Love cannot simply be phoned in. It must be outwardly demonstrated through meaningful and loving interactions. And the same is true for the dementia sufferer.

When I refer to quality time, I am referring to time when they receive your undivided attention and you are not busy managing or attending to other tasks. Dedicate special moments when you can sit quietly and try to understand their feelings, anticipate their concerns, and most importantly, reassure them that they are safe. Explain where they are living and who the people are who are caring for them. Explain that you live nearby and that you can be by their side in a matter of minutes. Give them your telephone number or tell them that the nurses would be happy to call you anytime that they would like to talk. Reassure them that their money is deposited safely in the bank and they can have it anytime that they like. Tell them that the doctors say that they are doing well and that they must continue to take care of themselves by taking their medicine. Remind them that they are intelligent.

- Tell them the stories of their life.

Recount stories of their personal and professional triumphs. Talk about their past. Become a storyteller. For Nan my recollections always begin and end in rural Ohio. The farm is always present during our time together, because I cannot look at Nan and not think of her farm. I share my memories of her barns and fields that look verdant and lush to the birds flying overhead. I tell her stories of Hereford cows, sheep, canning jars, and windmills. I describe the red glow of the workers' cigarettes as they gather at dusk after a long day of haying. Sometimes my stories sound like dreams or fairy tales that should begin with "once upon a time."

Often Nan looks at me in disbelief as I describe this magical place bursting with spring lilacs and autumn cattails. I describe the up-and-down motion of the handle on the ancient pump by the side of the house that still trickles sweet spring water. And together we ring the giant bell that cries out every mealtime. I know she doesn't often recognize that these stories belong to her. But she imagines this life, this far-off, wondrous place, much as a child who envisions herself like the princess in a fairy tale. And for a short time, inside this refuge, she is calm and relaxed. I will never know if my stories have triggered some distant memory, or if she feels the shelter of her beloved trees or hears the sound of the old iron gate when it introduced callers. If I am lucky, she might hear the wind calling her name through the distant woods reminding her that this magical place still lives deep inside her. It may belong to her, but I too find comfort in our visits to the old farm. And in the end, that is enough for both of us.

INSIGHTS

- Remember to provide a continual stream of love and reassurance to your loved one.
- Realize that although emotional security may be difficult to create for your loved one, you can increase the likelihood by implementing a few simple guidelines.
- Take time to tell your loved one the stories of their life. Speak of happy times when they were successful, strong, and confident.
- Monitor all individuals on your loved one's care team to ensure that they are always kind and supportive.
- Demonstrate physical love and affection each time you are with your loved one.
- Push your feelings to the side and buy a doll or stuffed animal that will provide comfort to your loved one.
- Remember to act as the voice for your loved one. Demonstrate that you will handle any problem that arises and take each of their concerns seriously.

16

HUMOR IS THE BEST MEDICINE

Laugh now, cry later.

—Erma Bombeck
The Grass Is Always Greener Over the Septic Tank

As a woman of a *certain age*, I can tell you with complete certainty that humor acts as a wonderful counterbalance to all of life's calamities. During difficult times, humor has been my friend and savior. It has been my reprieve and my sabbatical from worry and fear. Humor has lifted my burden so that I can lie down in the soft grass and ease my tired, aching shoulders. As I rest, joy playfully flickers down through the leaves in bright rays of sunshine. And when I am refreshed and heady with relief, I rise once again, brush myself off, and continue along my way, encouraged and invigorated.

When faced with the hard blows of life, we often don't allow ourselves to break down and laugh. Oh, it is fine to break down and cry or have a good weep, but to break down and laugh is often seen as taboo, insensitive, and unfeeling. Each of us has been given an incredible gift, a natural built-in medicine that we only elect to take in very small doses. When was the last time that you laughed so hard that you had tears in your eyes? When was the last time you allowed yourself to forget your caregiving problems and become lost inside a funny book or movie? My guess is that it has been far too long. Well to that I say, "Enough!"

We have all heard that laughter is good for what ails us. Studies prove that it diminishes pain, decreases stress levels, increases our immune system, and improves the quality of our lives. Oh yes, and it just plain feels good as it releases endorphins, those natural, feel-good hormones that give us a sense of well-being.[1] Humor also breeds hope and helps confirm our belief that we can make it through any situation. Laughter relaxes us so that we can regroup and begin again. If I had my way, the old adage would be, "A good belly laugh a day keeps the doctor away."

I know that there is nothing funny about a diagnosis of dementia. It feels like the end of all that is joyful and bright in the world. It signals the inevitable death of a personality and years of endless caregiving. It is a trap capable to pulling an entire family into a thick fog of black ether. It breeds worry and anxiety, and if you aren't careful, it can swallow you whole. But by now you know my anthem. You know that I believe that joy and happiness are possible despite the hardships of this disease. I believe that we have the power to stop looking through a lens of negativity and focus on the existence of courage and hope. And with this hope, joy is made possible.

If you are really honest with yourself, you will admit that caring for a dementia patient can put you in some very outrageous situations. It took me a long time to allow myself to see the comedy in many of the predicaments I found myself in, and even longer to not feel guilty for noticing them. Only after pushing aside my guilt have I been able to laugh at some of the ridiculous circumstances I have landed in while caring for Nan. Truthfully, she can be very funny. Her responses are often so comical and my attempts to gain her cooperation are so absurd, that I have no alternative but to laugh.

Nan, or as I sometimes think of her, Shecky Parsons, can parcel out her zingers and one-liners with lightning speed commensurate with any stand-up routine. For example, if my husband is late to take her for a ride, she'll say, "You're late, Sonny. Let's roll." If she doesn't like my perfume, she'll greet me with, "Hi, Stinky." If my husband asks her to do something that she has no interest in doing, she'll say, "You used to be such a nice boy." When she is mad or frustrated with me, she will say, "Hey dummy, hit the road." If she doesn't like her food, she will call it "slop," open her mouth, show it to me, and then squint her eyes as if trying to decide whether to spit it at me. Next she makes a kind of dramatic fake gagging noise before she swallows it down. And when she was first confined to a wheelchair, she turned an imaginary steering wheel and pushed an invisible gas pedal when she wanted to go faster.

The truth is that she can be very entertaining and frankly, hysterically funny.

One day when she first came to live near us, I arrived for my usual visit and asked her how she was doing. She replied, "Not good. I can't even go like this." She then raised both of her arms in the air. I said, "But you can go like that. You just did." To this she replied, "No I can't. I was just showing what I would like to be able to do if I was having a good day." The entire time she was speaking to me she was holding both arms above her head.

Nan used to have a problem with her neighbors who rode motorized scooters in the halls instead of traditional wheelchairs. Personally, I think that she was jealous. When they zoomed past her she would tell me to go and give them a ticket or shout out after them that they were over the speed limit. When I tried to explain to her that those poor people rode on scooters because they were unable to walk, she told me that I was wrong and that they just liked driving "fancy cars." I can still see her pumping her imaginary gas pedal in an attempt to overtake those imaginary speed demons.

No matter what situation you may find yourself in, there is always a small space available for laughter and humor. Sometimes I feel like I am a living testimony to the old adage, "If I don't laugh, I'll cry." I know that there is pathos behind each of the funny things that Nan says and does, a certain black humor. But like everything else in life, I am faced with a choice. I can either give into the sadness and remain perpetually miserable, or I can lighten up, realize that I can't control everything, and just roll with it.

One day I had the bright idea that instead of going through the rigmarole of trying to get her in and out of my car, I would simply push her wheel chair across the street for her scheduled doctor's appointment. After all it was only a few hundred yards. All went well on the way there, and we arrived to her appointment on time and in fine order. However, on our return trip it was as if a switch had been flicked. The minute her wheels hit the pavement she began screaming and she continued to scream the entire way through the parking lot, across the street and into her building. There was nothing physically wrong with her. She had just decided to scream. I tried to calm her down, but it was no use. And the harder I tried, the louder she screamed. And the more she screamed, the more I found it oddly funny. At one point I even considered joining in and believe me, I certainly wanted to. I was in a truly absurd and funny situation. Looking back I am surprised that no one stopped to question me, since I am sure it looked as if I was kidnapping a little white-haired, elderly woman. But then again, who uses a wheelchair as their getaway vehicle?

My mother was diagnosed with breast cancer in the 1990s, when she was living in Pacific Grove, California. I immediately flew out from Michigan to the community hospital where she was receiving treatment. Its cancer ward was phenomenal and was dedicated to healing the entire person through a variety of traditional and nontraditional methods. Their personnel saw the mind as a powerful healing tool. One of their nontraditional strategies was to encourage cancer sufferers to laugh every day. They had an enormous collection of humorous movies for their patients to watch. They believed that laughter had curative powers and aided the healing process. This was the first time that I had seen a traditional medical institution implement a program that incorporated the power of the mind into their treatment plan. I learned from their insight and remembered their wisdom when coping with Nan's condition.

Finding ways to tickle Nan's funny bone is not an easy task. As I mentioned earlier, Nan lost her ability to understand and see irony early in her disease, making it impossible for her to laugh at traditional jokes. This is why I rejoice when she finds an incident in her everyday life funny. I've seen her brought to tears over an odd comment or funny face. Typically the subject of her delight is the poor beleaguered nursing staff as they scurry around their central station. Granted, I am not usually in on the joke, but that is of no importance. I just enjoy seeing her happy and am pleased that she is still able to find situations funny. In this instance her humor feels organic, like a natural form of expression.

Since I cannot rely on the nursing staff to produce a hilarious floor show each day, I have accumulated a large video library containing funny movies and television comedy shows to help pick up the slack. I began with some of her favorites like Shirley Temple, Fred Astaire and Ginger Rogers, The Marx Brothers, Abbott and Costello, *The Lucy Show*, *Leave It to Beaver*, and *The Andy Griffith Show*. She and I have watched countless videos together, because I think that comedy is always better when shared with someone. What begins as a chuckle often turns into a belly laugh. Merriment always unites us and reinforces our strong bonds of trust and friendship. I hope that each time we laugh at the antics of Barney Fife her heart is made a bit lighter.

One afternoon when flipping through the television channels looking for a music program, we stopped for a brief moment on the cartoon show *Tom and Jerry*. I was surprised to see that she found these two very funny. I dared not move, in case I would break the spell. After a few minutes of watching poor Tom getting clobbered, she turned to me and said, "That kitty's going to get it." On the surface it may seem sad that such an intelligent woman was entertained by a child's cartoon. And yes, I could have decided to see it this way. But instead I chose to be grateful that she was happy, and I laughed at her charming response. This small sentence has become a maxim that my husband and I use when we see trouble on the horizon. "That kitty's going to get it" is a wonderful saying that always brings a smile to our faces and reminds us yet again that Nan is still in there.

As a caregiver, humor is also an effective tactic in my diversionary arsenal. After a long day with doctors or working with Nan, I love to read a funny book or watch a favorite comedy on television. I no longer like to watch sad dramas about dysfunctional families or doomed law cases. No, I'd much rather get lost between the words written by my dear old friend P. G. Wodehouse. He is my humor guru, the man who I cannot read in public because I may burst out laughing in a fit of hysteria or be forced to grope in my purse for tissues to dry my crying eyes. There is no way that I can read the adventures of Pongo Twistleton, Bertie Wooster, and anyone at the Drones Club and not laugh out loud. Mr. Wodehouse always lifts my spirits and is my comrade in comedy. As a card-carrying member of the P. G. Wodehouse Society, I realize that I am a bit biased, but I can't think of any situation in which his words would not force anyone to feel a bit more "Right Ho."

Let's face it. You can't feel sad or anxious when you are laughing. Humor embraces our entire being and dissolves disturbing emotions. It allows us to shift our perspective in order to view our situation from a different angle. It recharges our batteries and makes every obstacle seem less daunting. When my husband and I giggle over one of Nan's funny comments, we feel less overwhelmed by her disease and we view her and our family's situation in a better light.

We all know that dementia progresses over time. It speeds along, out of our control, each day adding new burdens for the caregiver. Consequently, we face serious concerns each day—mind-deadening concerns that can easily drain our sense of humor. Sometimes it feels disloyal and inappropriate to have any kind of fun. But it is important to understand that when we give into this sadness, we undermine every goal that we are working so hard to achieve.

Don't become a martyr to dementia. Being frustrated and miserable only stifles our energy and negatively impacts our interactions with our loved ones. Remember that your moods are contagious. Allow yourself to find the humor in your challenging and often ridiculous situations. Embrace a bit of nonsense every now and again. Work hard to uncover the absurdity and irony that lie behind each of life's situations. It is not wrong or disloyal to blow off a little steam and forget your problems for a short while. If you do, you will be better prepared to face the next inevitable challenge that dementia has in store for you.

No matter what you find funny, read it, watch it, do it, enjoy it. Let yourself go. Have a good laugh from time to time. Tell a joke. Go to a comedy club. Laugh with your children. I guarantee that you will instantly feel better and that the hills before you will seem less steep. As a fellow caregiver, I am giving you permission to have fun and see the humor in the amusing things that your loved one says and does. After all, we are not laughing at them, we are laughing with them. And as Mark Twain so aptly put it, "The human race has only one really effective weapon and that is laughter. The moment it arises, all your irritations and resentments slip away, and the sunny spirit takes their place."[2]

INSIGHTS

- Laughter truly is the best medicine. It has been proven to diminish pain, decrease stress levels, and boost our immune systems.
- Give up the guilt. Allow yourself to laugh at the ridiculous situations that you land in while caring for your loved one.
- Recognize the humor in your loved one's funny responses.
- Create a collection of humorous videos that you can share with your loved one.

- Take time to do whatever lightens your load. Read funny books. Watch funny movies. Spend time with friends who make you laugh.
- Look to your loved one's past in order to find ways to introduce humor into their everyday life. What movies or comedians did they find funny? What was their favorite comedy television program?
- Lighten up. After all, it is better to laugh than it is to cry.

17

THE CAREGIVER

It's not enough to have lived. We should be determined to live for something.

May I suggest that it be creating joy for others, sharing what we have for the betterment of personkind, bringing hope to the lost and love to the lonely.

—Leo Buscaglia

Do you know that you are a hero? You have incredible inner strength and possess the mightiest courage. You willingly added the burdens of another to the load that you bear, a feat that few others would attempt. You are a brave star illuminating the darkness of night. You chose to rise above your personal needs and looked uncertainty and sadness square in the eye. You are a healer, a mender, a bell ringer calling forth your divinity to be shared with the world. You were selected for this reason. You are the difference maker, the fixer-of-things, and the architect of metamorphosis. You are a spirit-filled vessel scattering seeded blessings throughout the universe.

Caring for another individual changes who you are and how you view the entire world. I have never had a child but have been told countless times that being responsible for another human being, another precious life, is the most fulfilling and scary adventure that we can experience. It is a blessing filled with immeasurable responsibilities and a great many worries. Of course the sad difference between parenthood and caregiving is the eventual outcome. With parenthood comes hope for future possibilities, while caring for a dementia patient leads to sadness and inevitable loss. But both are derivatives of love, a love strong enough to transcend a rocking cradle or a quiet bedside. Either way they leave us, one to venture out into the world and the other to rest eternally upon a quiet hillside.

Caring for Nan has shown me traits about myself that I never knew I possessed, ones that for a lifetime had lain dormant. The act of caregiving remolded me like clay upon a potter's wheel. It has made me a better person, for I came to see the world around me with fresh eyes. What was once common is now extraordinary. What was trivial is now a blessing. What was a frustration is now a victory. What was anger has been transformed into love, much like the appearance of tiny, chartreuse leaves that burst forth after a harsh and bitter winter. Caring for Nan has shined a light into the dark corners of my life and shown me what is really important. It has forced me to reprioritize my goals and walk a different path. Was there a price? Yes, my strength was gained with the sacrifice of time and hard work, repeated again and again until all my worries and bitterness were ground to dust.

For one moment I would like you to forget about your loved one. Think only of yourself, the caregiver who is often underappreciated or overlooked. I want you to take stock of everything in your life from your stress level, to your relationships, to your health. I want you to consider bestowing the same tender care and concern that you give to your loved one onto yourself. Attend to your immediate needs and set long-term goals for your life. Follow passionate pursuits and have fun. Make your mark upon the world. I want you to honestly assess your life and give yourself permission to make whatever changes are necessary to lead a healthy and fulfilling life.

You might be asking, "How do you know that I am not doing that already?" I know because I have walked in your shoes. I know with complete certainty that you have placed your needs on the back burner so that you can pour all your energy into caring for your loved one. It didn't start out that way. You certainly never intended to push your own requirements to one side and neglect your own personal happiness and well-being. But it happened, gradually. Over time the needs of the patient took over your life, like weeds invading an untended garden.

You take your loved one to the doctor, but tend to put your own health concerns on the back burner. You worry over their wardrobe and personal grooming, when you could use a new outfit or a day at the salon. You urge them to eat a balanced diet, while you grab a quick hamburger from a fast-food restaurant and eat it in your car. You sit by their side watching them nap after you laid awake the previous night worrying over unsolvable problems. Just because you willingly decided to care for someone you love deeply, does not mean that there are not times when it is all-consuming and draining. Many days I have been weary beyond belief and wonder how I will find the strength to do what needs to be accomplished.

When you are a caregiver of a dementia patient, no matter where you go or what you do, their situation is there with you, the proverbial elephant in the room. Whether you are involved in another activity or trying to accomplish a nonrelated task, it is always there, niggling at you, distracting you from what you are trying to accomplish. The patient's needs are never far from your mind.

For me this increased as Nan's condition deteriorated and my stress level rose. As her agitation, emotional outbursts, and episodes of wandering increased, I found it more difficult to relax and take a mental reprieve from my role as a caregiver. This was particularly difficult for the first six months after she moved to Virginia—a time when all of her symptoms were escalating at breakneck speed—and ended up being the worst period in my caregiving experience. I was constantly receiving calls from her memory unit because she completely refused to cooperate with the staff. Nan would take everything off her shelves and drop them onto the floor. She even managed to pull her television off its stand. She would steal items belonging to other residents. She was loud, belligerent, and at times scary because she still had the physical strength to put up a fight. It was almost impossible to *convince* her to do anything. These difficult days led to the creation of my Moment by Moment technique.

One problem was particularly difficult for me to handle. Nan refused to let the nurses' aides change her diapers. Consequently, they would call me and ask me to come over and try to reason with her. Sometimes it took an hour to get through to her. When it was over, I would be left so emotionally and physically drained that I would sit quietly for some time in order to regain my equilibrium. It was during these dark days when I made the decision that I needed to toss my needs into the mix. I needed to schedule time when I could enjoy a world that was not crazy and spinning out of control.

I want to encourage you to do the same. I want you to put your needs first from time to time. Yes, I said first. Learn from my mistakes so that you don't become weary and exhausted. After all, when we are on an airplane, they instruct us to put on our oxygen mask before helping others. The same applies in the caregiving situation. If you are stressed, tired, and physically shattered, you will be of no constructive use to anyone. You must take care of yourself.

But I must warn you that this step cannot be taken without feeling guilty. It happens to every caregiver and I think it is part of the job description: *When not spending every waking moment focusing on the immediate needs of their loved one, the caregiver will feel ashamed and guilt ridden.* See, there it is in writing, a rule stating that once you become a caregiver you must forfeit any desire for personal happiness.

Well, I say that it is time that you and I rewrite this rule. I say that you should stop being so hard on yourself and think of it this way: How can you create joy and happiness in the life of another individual when you are emotionally depleted and not nurturing your own zest for life?

As I have said before, caregiving is a tough business. You have to be on your toes, ready to hit the next curve ball out of the park. You need to be up to the challenge. I don't care if you have to schedule time off and hire an aide while you relax, you absolutely must find a way to attend to your personal needs.

Nan spent the five years before her devastating heart attack caring for her elderly, invalid husband. She kept him at home on the farm and worked tirelessly preparing meals and caring for him physically. Once a week a county nurse would come to help bathe him, but otherwise Nan was on her own. She placed a hospital bed in the dining room and became her husband's full-time caregiver. She absolutely refused to place him in a nursing home and try as we might, there was nothing that any of us could have said or done that would have changed her mind. In the clarity of hindsight I wish that we had insisted a little harder, but I know that our efforts would have fallen on deaf ears. Nothing could have stopped Nan from honoring her wedding vows to cherish her husband *in sickness and in heath*, but unwittingly she was placing herself in jeopardy.

Nan followed the old definition of caregiving to the letter and consequently neglected important aspects of her own life. Her dental health declined. She chose to ignore occasional chest pains that occurred when she overexerted herself. In the end, she paid a very high price for being a loyal and fervent wife. As I mentioned earlier, medical professionals believe that her heart attack precipitated her subsequent dementia. I think of this often and try to imagine a different scenario in which Nan took care of herself, never had her heart attack, and her dementia never occurred. How different all of our lives would be. Nan's story is a caregiving cautionary tale for anyone who may be following in her foot-steps. Like Nan, you may think that this could never happen to you, but it can and it does every day.

And if that doesn't convince you, think of it this way. I am certain that your loved one would not want you to be a sacrificial lamb laid on the altar of their dementia. No, they would want you to be healthy and still enjoy your life. I know that they would want you to remain a participant in the world around you, spend time with friends, and share in all the wonderful aspects of life that they are no longer able to enjoy. So if you won't do it for yourself, consider doing it for them.

CARING FOR THE CAREGIVER

- Take care of yourself physically. Schedule regular doctors' visits and annual screening examinations. It is incredibly easy to overlook your own needs when you are coping with the demands of caregiving. Time can pass very quickly when you are embroiled in the physical and mental needs of another person. Schedule your doctor and dentist appointments in advance, mark them in your calendar, and don't let anything or anyone cause you to cancel them.
- Schedule time away from the patient. Give yourself permission to take regular breaks by building time off into your caregiving schedule. Hire assistance if necessary or ask family members to help out one day a week. Consider finding a local adult day-care center that has experience dealing with memory-impaired individuals. Go to lunch with a friend. Take a class. Participate in an activity that brings you pleasure. Plan a yearly vacation to a relaxing destination. A change of scenery will help keep your responsibilities in perspective. If you are afraid to leave your loved one at home, find a facility that offers short-term respite stays. And most importantly, keep

reminding yourself that there is a big, wide, wonderful world outside
the parameters of caregiving.

- Accept help when it is offered. Let others show their love for you by
  allowing them to spend time with your loved one. This was particularly difficult for me. I saw Nan as my responsibility and didn't want
  to pass my burden onto anyone else. I felt that I had to be in control
  of everything that happened to her. It took me quite some time to
  realize that my friends were sincere. They genuinely wanted to help.
  Once I agreed to let them sit with Nan on occasion, it was beneficial
  for both Nan and me. I got a short reprieve while Nan was able to
  meet and enjoy new people.

- Enlist the help of your entire family. If your relatives live locally,
  don't leave their visits to chance. Develop a monthly schedule so that
  they make regular, planned visits to your loved one. This affords you
  predetermined time away from your duties so that you can schedule
  time for activities and appointments. If you know in advance when
  your loved one will have visitors, you will be able to maximize your
  free time. If your family members live out of town, ask them when
  they plan to come for a visit. This may be a good time for you to
  schedule that much-needed vacation or just to have a luxurious, care-
  free week.

- Pay close attention to your moods and feelings. Research has shown
  that 30–40 percent of individuals who provide care for someone with
  dementia suffer from depression.[1] Depression in caregivers can man-
  ifest into a variety of symptoms—for example, a change in eating
  habits, feeling tired all the time, loss of interest in people or activities
  that once brought you pleasure, a change in sleeping patterns, ongo-
  ing physical symptoms that do not respond to treatment, such as
  headaches, digestive disorders, and chronic pain.[2] If you are experiencing any of these symptoms, seek professional help from a doctor
  or counselor. Help can also be found through local and national
  Alzheimer's and dementia support organizations. Stay attuned to
  your feelings and don't feel guilty or selfish if you decide to seek
  help. Be kind to yourself and know that you are not alone. Many
  individuals in your situation have benefited from professional
  support.

- Devote time to pursue your passions. Even though you are busy, take
  time to enjoy your favorite hobbies and interests. Find ways to

channel your creative energy or learn something new. Take French lessons or that pottery class that you have talked about for years. Unleash your inner artist. Be courageous. Create something beautiful or read a new poem each day. Nourish your soul with whatever you find extraordinary and meaningful.

- Write in a daily journal. Take time each day to write down your concerns and feelings. This will allow you to stay in touch with your authentic self. Research shows that journaling reduces stress and provides an outlet to freely express thoughts and feelings. It provides a neutral forum in which we can vent and resolve feelings of conflict with individuals or our current situation.[3] By writing about our problems, we are better able to pinpoint their source and find appropriate solutions.

- Exercise regularly. As a caregiver it is imperative that you find time in your schedule for regular exercise. It not only clears your head and boosts your spirits, but also has been proven to reduce stress levels.

- Lighten you load by taking advantage of eligible services that are available to your loved one—for example, financial support, county nursing assistance, Meals on Wheels, and Medicare-provided home health services.

- Seek spiritual guidance. If you are feeling overwhelmed, consider making an appointment to talk to your pastor, rabbi, or priest. Ask that others remember you in their prayers.

- Make exciting plans for the future. Schedule pleasurable events in the future so that you have something to anticipate. Buy tickets to a play or musical performance that will be appearing in your town. My husband and I are fond of chamber music, so each year we purchase season tickets through our local Chamber Music Society. It is our guarantee that each month we will experience an evening filled with our favorite music.

- Pamper yourself. Treat yourself to activities that reduce your stress. Spend a day at a health or beauty spa. Watch a favorite movie. Soak in a warm bubble bath. Schedule a full body massage. Do whatever relaxes you and feels luxurious.

When you became a caregiver you answered a calling. Learn to honor yourself in the same way that you honor your loved one. For when you are refreshed and at peace, it is as if all your doors and windows have been flung wide open. It is then that love and compassion can pass freely in and out of your life and you will have energy to shower onto your loved one.

Because after all, no one deserves it more than you.

May you become soothed by the song of the meadowlark, comforted by the warm streams of afternoon sunshine, find relief as tender as a falling autumn leaf, and catch the peace that sails on a gentle ocean wave. And in the end, I hope that the blessings that you have bestowed on your loved one keep lifting you higher and higher, until the orbiting stars and you merge into one.

INSIGHTS

- Give yourself credit for taking on the enormous challenge of caregiving.
- Focus on the strength that you have gained by being a caregiver.
- Take stock of your life. Gauge your stress level, happiness, relationships, and health.
- Create time when you will not allow yourself to think about your caregiving responsibilities.
- Schedule days off from your caregiving duties. Enlist the help of friends and family to visit your loved one while you are away.
- Step back from the situation. Take the focus off your loved one and allow yourself to celebrate all that is joyful and wonderful in your life.
- Rewrite the traditional definition of *caregiving*.
- Don't become a martyr to dementia. In the end, you will pay a heavy price.
- Take care of yourself physically. Eat healthy foods, exercise, and *never* postpone your annual doctors' visits or screenings.
- Plan an adventure in the future so that you have something delightful to anticipate.
- Monitor your moods and feelings. If you are feeling helpless or depressed, seek medical attention from a doctor or counselor.
- Make time to pursue your passions and interests.
- Make sure that you are taking full advantage of all the eligible services that are available to your loved one.
- Remember to nourish your spirit.

- Take time to pamper yourself. Schedule a massage, manicure, or spa treatment.
- Be attuned to the reality that there is life beyond your caregiving experience.

18

THE BUSINESS OF DEMENTIA

For every minute spent organizing, an hour is earned.

—Anonymous

There is more to being a caregiver than meets the eye. Behind all of my daily responsibilities lay mountains of paperwork and tough decisions. As Nan's president and chief financial officer, I know that my actions impact every component of her life. I manage her money, pay her bills, handle her correspondence, and track her medical progress. Without careful management on my part, Nan would not be able to maximize her life physically or financially. In order for her to have the joy-filled life that I have planned for her, I have to take my responsibilities seriously, be organized, and prepare for the future.

By definition, dementia is uncontrollable. It is complex and overwhelming as it blazes a trail through every aspect for your life. When a loved one is struck down by dementia, your world becomes a series of *mights*. Your loved one *might* get worse, or they *might* remain stable. They *might* have enough money to last the remainder of their life, or they *might* become insolvent. They *might* be able to continue to live on their own, or they *might* need to move into a nursing facility. As you know, the worries or *mights* come at you like a fast-moving conveyor belt. As I have told you before, the only way that I found to slow the speed of these negative feelings is to take control over the controllables.

To the right of my desk stands a large, built-in bookcase filled with souvenirs from my life. The shelves hold incoming and outgoing correspondence; an old, Paris airplane boarding pass; a picture postcard my father sent me in 1964 when he was on a business trip in London; and bright sticky notes penned with newly discovered quotes waiting to be transferred into a little leather book I keep solely for this purpose. This clutter represents my endangered pleasures. In a world where almost a million written pages can be held on a memory stick the size of a gum wrapper, I still use a pen and paper to annotate little inspirations that cross my path each day. Yes, I know that I am a bit of a dinosaur, but I still love the feel of a pen in my hand as it glides across smooth, cool paper, and the sound the book spine makes each time I open it.

In my bookcase I have dedicated one complete shelf to the business side of Nan's life. It consists of a neat row of three-ringed binders, clearly labeled so that I can access information quickly. I have everything that I need right at my fingertips. When I first began caring for Nan, I organized her records in a traditional filing system, which was an effective storage solution for documents that I rarely needed, like birth and marriage certificates, wills, and insurance policies. But in a crisis, like when I needed to hurry to the hospital or nursing facility, I found shuffling thorough files to locate emergency information maddening and inefficient. So I set up a dual filing system. I created a set of binders to hold Nan's current and pertinent information, and used my traditional files for older medical information and records that I rarely utilize.

This system has been an efficient, convenient, and effective way to track all the details of Nan's life. Now when I receive an emergency call or am preparing for a doctor's visit or care meeting, I simply select the appropriate notebook and I am out the door. And the best part is that if for some reason I am unavailable, my husband knows where to find any information that he might need in an emergency. This system has proven to be a real time-saver for both of us.

Since Nan's care plan is constantly being altered, it can be difficult to remember each small change. My husband may even be unaware of the most recent doctor's orders. But by referring to the appropriate binder he can be up-to-speed in a matter of seconds. He has access to Nan's current information so that he can make wise and informed decisions. Two years ago when we were leaving the country for three weeks, my sister-in-law stayed in our home in order to look after Nan. Both she and I were able to relax knowing that in case of emergency, she would have no difficulty locating Nan's current medical and insurance records.

Setting up your system only requires a few three-ring binders and a small amount of your time. When a binder becomes full or when information has become outdated, I rotate records into a traditional permanent file. I am confident that once you have created your notebook library, you will find that it is an easy way to track your loved one's progress. I think you will wonder how you ever got along without it.

BINDER LIBRARY

The first binder I created is entitled NAN. This is where I keep important legal and medical information regarding Nan. It is my *go-to* book, the one that I grab in an emergency situation. It holds the following information:

- Copies of her Social Security card, Medicare card, insurance cards, and photo identification. Be sure to include copies of all your loved one's benefit cards—for example, supplementary insurance cards, drug prescription card, Medicare card, Medicaid card, and Medicare Part D card.
- A copy of her advanced directive or Do Not Resuscitate order.
- Her complete medical history including her medical conditions, chronic diseases, major illnesses, and surgeries with their appropriate dates and locations.
- A copy of her Durable Power of Attorney and Health Care Power of Attorney.
- A master calendar where I track her recent and upcoming doctors' appointments and meetings.
- A list of her current medications, their dosages, and the date they were prescribed. Be sure to include any PRN medications that your loved one has been prescribed—for example, aspirin, Ativan, acetaminophen, nebulizer treatments, and cough medicines.
- A copy of Nan's current eyeglass prescription.
- An updated contact list of family, doctors, facility, facility personnel, and friends.

The INSURANCE binders are where I keep claims and Explanation of Benefits (EOB) forms that are sent from Nan's insurance companies.

I have a separate binder for each company that insures her, including Medicare. I receive electronic notifications from her insurance companies via e-mail when a new EOB is available. I then print it and file it in the appropriate binder in descending order so that the most current claim is on top. Electronic services are available from most major insurance companies. This system makes it easy to match incoming medical bills against insurance payouts and deductibles. I never pay a medical bill without making sure that the amount billed matches the appropriate EOB.

The DOCTORS binder has a section for each physician who cares for Nan. I file the List of Services paperwork that we receive at the end of each of her visits under the appropriate doctor's tab. I utilize this information when reconciling insurance claims and keeping track of the dates of her various diagnoses, infections, and illnesses.

The TEST RESULTS binder is partitioned into sections for blood work, scans, biopsies, X-rays, and surgical explanations.

The MONEY binder is where I keep copies of Nan's bank statements, retirement accounts, and portfolio summaries. You will appreciate your organization when tax season rolls around. Keep in mind that some medical expenses may qualify as allowable tax deductions. Contact your accountant to answer all of your tax questions.

It is also imperative to keep accurate and timely records when you are managing another individual's earnings and expenditures. No matter how small, document every financial outlay that you make on behalf of your loved one. This is your personal insurance in case other family members or future heirs question your actions. This ensures that you will have a complete account of every penny that you have spent while caring for the patient. Even family members who love one another and get along well can change when there is money at stake. Keeping accurate records will avoid any future misunderstandings or unjustified accusations. You may even consider purchasing an accounting ledger or computer program that will allow you to accurately track every dollar you outlay.

In addition, I constantly reassess Nan's financial portfolio to ensure that I am maximizing her earning potential so she will have adequate funds to pay her expenses in the future. I make it a point to keep enough liquid capital to pay her expenses for three months. This serves as my buffer against any unforeseen contingencies. The amount of cash that you elect to have on hand depends on your loved one's financial situation, their monthly expenses, and their total asset valuation.

In the CARE MEETINGS binder I track all the information that is provided during my bimonthly meetings with the staff at Nan's nursing facility. I chart her vital statistics, weight, blood sugar levels, and any behavioral issues that have arisen since the prior meeting. I also annotate my specific requests or concerns so that I can effectively follow up with specific accountable individuals.

As with any filing system, the key to success is to keep your records up-to-date. I have made a personal commitment to file new information in a timely manner. This ensures that I am prepared for any possible emergency. Don't put your filing off until later, because a filing system is only helpful if it is kept current. Remember, you may need vital information sooner than you think. The bottom line is: Be prepared.

As is often the case with dementia, Nan reached a point when it was no longer safe for her to live on her own. First, we tried to figure out a way that she could live with one of us if we hired outside help. It didn't take long for this solution to be taken off the table. Since she had never fully recovered from her broken hip, neither of our homes were equipped to handle Nan's physical limitations. Also the cost of twenty-four-hour care made this option cost prohibitive. We had no other choice but to place Nan in a long-term care facility.

This was not an easy decision for us to make. In fact, it was heart wrenching. We knew the lengths to which Nan had gone to keep her husband at home. But we had to be realistic. We had to step back from the situation and become pragmatic. Nan needed to be in a safe environment that was equipped to deal with her erratic behavior and physical limitations. She needed assistance with every aspect of her life, assistance that we were just not able to provide.

We also had to take into account that Nan is a very social person. She loves being around people and interacting with others. Forcing her to live in one of our homes would in essence be starving her of the multidimensional social interactions that she would enjoy in a more active setting. We knew that Nan would be happier if she could interact with a wide variety of people throughout her day. We also thought that a more diverse social setting would help keep her mind active.

So we began our hunt. My husband and I visited no fewer than fifteen local care facilities before making a final decision. We investigated each of our options thoroughly because we did not want to move Nan multiple times. Moving is an enormous adjustment for you and me, so can you imagine how overwhelming it is for an individual who is cognitively impaired. We became investigators who evaluated each facet of every facility that we toured. Here is the list of factors and key information we learned during our search:

- Make sure that the nursing home and current administrator are both licensed.
- Google the institution that you are considering. Read the reviews and see if it has received any negative press reports in the media.
- Ask to see copies of the facility's most recent state inspection reports. In what areas were they delinquent? In what areas did they excel?
- Trust your first impressions. Is the facility well maintained? Are the grounds neat and tidy? Do you smell an unpleasant odor when you enter the building? If you smell urine, you know immediately that residents are not being toileted properly and that workers are not disposing of soiled undergarments properly. Does the lobby appear clean and organized?
- Does the facility appear safe? Are the hallways free of clutter? Are the exits clearly marked? Are visitors asked to check in before entering the facility? Is the front door staffed during the hours that the doors are unlocked? What time do they lock the main doors at night? What is their evening and weekend visiting policy? Do they conduct fire drills? What are their emergency procedures? Do they have a generator to power the facility during a power outage?
- Be sure to understand all costs associated with living at the facility. The truth is that each of us must live within our means. Although all nursing facilities are expensive, some facilities require a large up-front fee for a resident to become a part of the community. Also ask for a list of what products and services are included in the monthly rent. This is especially important if you are investigating an assisted living facility. Often institutions charge according to the level of care that the resident requires. For example, if

your loved one is able to dress and bathe themselves, the fees could be substantially lower than if they need assistance with these activities. In Nan's assisted living facility, they offered five levels of care that became progressively more expensive.

- Are there levels of care available within the community? Plan ahead. Even though your loved one may be able to function beautifully in an assisted living situation today, remember that dementia is a progressive disease. So if possible, choose a community where they can progress into a memory or nursing unit should the need arise. Make certain that residents already living in the community are moved to the top of all waiting lists and do not have to compete with outside individuals when seeking placement in these critical-care units.

- Are potential residents interviewed as a part of the application process? This is especially pertinent if your loved one is moving into an assisted living facility. Administrators want to make sure that they can live fairly independently with only minimal help and supervision.

- Is there a designated area for family and friends to visit with your loved one?

- Does the facility conduct thorough background checks on its entire staff?

- Does the staff seem friendly and helpful?

- Does the facility have a high staff turnover?

- Ask about staffing ratios. Or in other words, investigate the number of nurses and aides in relation to the number of residents. This is a critical factor when considering a home for your loved one. You want to ensure that there is always adequate staff to provide the care your loved one requires. States have strict laws governing these ratios for nursing facilities. However, in most states there are no such guidelines for assisted living facilities. This is a critical distinction when considering residential alternatives. Do your homework. Investigate the guidelines in your state so that you can make educated comparisons. Realize that these numbers are simply guidelines and are only the minimum staffing numbers required by law. During my search I encountered many facilities with higher staffing ratios in order to provide exemplary care. They do exist, but you have to work hard to find them. Ask about staffing ratios on nights, weekends, and holidays. Is the same level of care given to the residents regardless of the time of day or day of the week?

- Ask which hospital serves the facility. Is it highly rated and equipped with the latest medical services and technologies?
- Pay close attention to the facility's current residents. Are they well groomed? Is everyone neatly dressed, or are they sitting around in their bedclothes? Is their hair combed and brushed? Are the men's faces shaved? Do their clothes appear clean and unsoiled? Notice where the bulk of the residents are located. Are the majority lying in bed in their rooms or relegated to sit in the hallways, or are they sitting together peacefully in a common area?
- Ask if your loved one can keep their private physician or if they have to utilize a facility doctor. Inquire what doctors regularly visit the facility. Is there a dedicated physician who attends to the needs of all the residents? If so, how often do they visit? Ask if podiatrists, optometrists, and dentists pay regular visits to the facility. Often, doctors who visit nursing facilities do not have an actual office in which they see patients. This can make it difficult to investigate their reviews and obtain customer feedback. Once you have the name of the facility physician, investigate them online to look for any complaints submitted to the American Medical Association.
- Ask about the facility's regularly scheduled activities. Do they take their residents to local stores and musical performances? Do they have monthly birthday celebrations? Do outside performers come in and entertain the residents? Do they conduct sing-alongs? Do local organizations like the Veteran's Administration pay visits to honor veteran residents? Do they have a gardening program? Do they have movie night? Do residents have access to Wi-Fi and Internet? Do pets come and visit? What games do they offer?
- Is there a garden or patio area where you can sit outside with your loved one? As you know, this was a very important requirement when selecting each of Nan's facilities. It was imperative that she have a place to enjoy fresh air and nature.
- Is there a nutritionist on site? Ask to look at the current month's menu plan. Ask if you can make arrangements to come for a noon or evening meal. What time are meals served? Is the dining room

clean and quiet? How do they handle food substitutions if a resident does not like what is being served? Do they offer diabetic and heart-healthy menus? Do they provide afternoon and evening snacks? Visit the dining room at mealtime to see if residents are receiving the help that they need to enjoy their food. Are they being encouraged to finish their meal? If residents are not eating, are they offered help or an alternative entrée? Is there adequate water provided at each place setting?

- How often do they monitor the resident's vital signs? How often are residents weighed?
- How frequently are residents bathed? Does the facility have shower seats and beds for the residents?
- Does the facility have an in-house hairdresser?
- How often are the residents hydrated and encouraged to drink water?

Even after you have conducted your thorough investigation, there is one more thing that you should do before making your final decision. If you want to see what really goes on at different times of the day, drop in unannounced. Don't call in advance or tell them you are coming. Just walk up to the front desk and ask to be escorted through the facility. I've always considered this to be the true litmus test.

Once you find a safe and loving home for your loved one, I must ask a favor of you. One that I know you will do willingly. I ask that you always remember to be kind to those who toil each day to care for the one you love. Theirs is not an easy job. On the contrary, it is often thankless and underpaid. Yet, they elect to wake each morning, leave their homes, and care for those who cannot care for themselves. They lift. They bathe. They soothe. They ache. Having known hundreds of caregivers who have tenderly cared for Nan, I am convinced that their vocation is the answer to an inner calling, a divine command to make the world a better place. Honor those who give of themselves each day to help your loved one. Let's repay them with gratitude and respect.

Most facility policies state that care workers cannot receive money from residents or their families. This means that we have to find creative ways to offer our thanks. Begin by putting your kind thoughts and kudos in writing. It doesn't matter if you pick up your pen, or sit at your keyboard, take the time to document a job well done by notifying the appropriate supervisors and administrators. In the often thankless world of nursing care, this can mean a great deal emotionally and financially. This small gesture could make all the difference during their quarterly review.

Your show of appreciation need not be grand. Bring the nurses a bouquet of flowers that are blooming in your garden. Place them in a mason jar with a tag that simply says, "Thank you." Bake three dozen cookies and place them in the staff lounge. Buy a large box of chocolates that can be enjoyed by all the employees. And of course there are those two tiny words that can never be underestimated, "Thank you."

When Nan was living in her first facility, twice a year my husband and I threw a pizza party for the entire staff. We scheduled them late in the afternoon between the day and evening shifts so that most of the staff would be able to attend. This was a relatively inexpensive gesture. Pizza companies advertise frequent specials and many offer pies for half price on designated days of the week. Be sure to get approval from the administrator before spreading the word, and always remember to purchase a few extra pizzas so that the night crew can enjoy a slice during their break or midnight meal.

The gift of gratitude need not be wrapped in gold or set with jewels to be valued by its recipient. Regardless of our standing or position, each of us has so much to be thankful for that we should leave the ground behind us covered with good wishes. Whether bestowed by kings or humble folks like you and me, gratitude has the power to move mountains and positively alter any situation. It facilitates cooperation and peace. It transforms upheaval into harmony. It is the alchemy that spins indifference into love.

INSIGHTS

- Do not wait to get organized.
- Create a filing system that is easily accessible and understood by everyone helping with caregiving responsibilities.
- Keep accurate and impeccable records of every expenditure that you make on behalf of your loved one.
- Create a binder containing all immediate medical and financial information that you might need in an emergency.

- Prepare for the future by closely monitoring and investing your loved one's financial portfolio.
- Communicate with other family members and develop a plan for the day your loved one passes on. This will save you from having to make emotional decisions during a very difficult time.
- Never pay a medical bill that does not match the EOB from your loved one's insurance company.
- If you think that your loved one's insurance has been incorrectly processed, do not hesitate to make inquiries.
- Keep track of all medications and medical tests administered to your loved one.
- If your loved one lives in a facility, take the time to prepare for your regular care meetings. Create an agenda of the topics that you would like to cover regarding your loved one's health and happiness.
- When considering a facility for your loved one, conduct a detailed and thorough investigation.
- Think ahead. If it looks like your loved one is going to need the care offered in a nursing facility, begin your investigation today.
- Remember that you are the mouthpiece for your loved one. Always remember to express your deep gratitude to all those who provide them with loving care.

19

GOING HOME

When he shall die,
Take him and cut him out in little stars,
And he will make the face of heaven so fine
That all the world will be in love with night,
And pay no worship to the garish sun.

—William Shakespeare
Romeo and Juliet

Deep within the tradition of Irish storytelling lays a mythical land off the west coast of Ireland called *Hy-Brasil*, or the *Isle of the Blest*. This Celtic paradise is home to souls who have passed on and exists "beyond all dreams, where all year round, the fruits hang bright and the flowers bloom in the meadows green. Wild honey drips from forest trees" with "endless stocks of meadow and wine. No illness comes from across the seas, nor death, nor pain, nor sad decline. The light and splendors all increase each day in this Golden Land of Youth."[1] If true, it is my hope that when each boat arrives at the island's shore, those who have suffered most will be among the first to disembark. My prayer is that they were made whole once again during this sacred crossing.

I've heard dementia described as the long goodbye and this is undeniably true. Slowly we watch the physical and mental capacities of someone we love drift away until they have been stripped clean to the bone. It is a wretched, heart-ripping, howling-at-the-moon kind of sad that steals souls before our eyes like a banshee that screams in the darkness. It rearranges the tiny molecules that hold a family together. It reassigns the roles that we have played for a lifetime; mother becomes daughter, daughter becomes mother. It is like watching someone slip into a dream while they are still awake.

I know that the day is fast approaching when I will lose Nan. I know this to be true because everything that I do for her carries the soft whisper of *bon voyage.* Each day, a piece of her seems to break free and float away. I know that I am in a race against time, so I remain busy collecting memories for the day when she will be gone. Since the time I have to love her is dwindling, I am more determined than ever to enjoy her *moment by moment.* Nan and I have entered into that odd time of preparing, she for a journey and me bracing myself for the time when all the pieces of her will have blown away like scattered seeds from a late summer milkweed.

Like everything else in the ambiguous world of dementia, being prepared is the best way to cope with the uncertainty. Speak to family members now and plan for the day when your loved one goes home. Make all the painful decisions now so that your burden will be lighter when you get the inevitable phone call.

Many years ago when my father was losing his long battle with cancer, I would pass his room at night and see a chink of light shining from beneath his closed door. In those quiet moments when all the distractions of the world were stilled, I was forced to face the truth. I could no longer pretend. He was not going to get well. I was going to lose him. Even though I never interrupted his privacy, in my mind I saw him sitting on the edge of his bed, shoulders low and his head in his hands. I could not quite make out if he was praying or crying—perhaps both— but I knew that during those dark hours, he too could no longer pretend. He knew what I knew. I have never spoken of these moments with anyone. They are too intimate to be tainted by words. But it was through a closed door, alone in the middle of the night, that I understood for certain that I was losing my father.

You are grace alive, working each day to elevate your life and those whom you have sought to help. Unfortunately, everything in the Moment by Moment technique leads up to a departing. Hopefully by now you have realized that the joy you created was not just for your loved one, but also for you. It was a gift that you unwittingly gave to yourself. So when that sad day of reckoning arrives and all your accounts are settled, I am certain that you will have no regrets. You will remember how hard you tried to create sunshine to brighten rainy days and create shade when the glare from the sun was too harsh. I do not know how, but after your loved one moves on, I know that they will be made aware of your kindness and their spirit will cry *thank you*. They will see your tender care as a divine benediction. I have no proof of this. You will just have to trust me. Because sometimes you have to have faith to believe that everything will be made right, even when you are standing outside your father's closed door in the middle of the night.

Just think of it. After they leave us they will be whole again, restored in mind and body. It is we who will be left to begin again, for they will have taken their place among the nightly stars shining forever in a mighty blaze of eternal joy.

Stones signify transformation and the continuation of life, a memory talisman. Whenever I visit a grave I always place a stone on the marker. Like my love of the soil, my urge to gather stones is primal and innate. Ancient wood resin becomes amber. Limestone becomes marble. Calcium and iron become jade. Years ago I carried home a small stone from a cottage in Chiddingstone, England, where my parents had spent the early days of their marriage. I placed this stone atop their marker in honor of the sweet dreams of their youth. Other times I have brought stones from the houses where I have lived, houses that they never visited. I bring them stones to prove that they are not forgotten and in appreciation of the life I was given when they rescued me. By now I am sure that the stones I brought are buried as deep as my roots in the beloved Ohio soil.

But for Nan, I want it to be different. I don't want to wait until I visit her on some distant hillside before I begin gathering her stones. I want to pay homage to her now, today, while I can still look in her blue, crinkled eyes. So each day I bring her my stones, stones in the guise of love, so that they may be intermingled with her heart and not placed atop cold granite carved with her name. Each day I bring a new offering. Yesterday it was *joy*. Today it was *dignity*. Tomorrow it will be *gratitude*.

To each of us a ticket is given, a date and a time stamped so faintly we cannot read it, whispered so softly that we can't hear it. When our train is called, we have no choice but to be on the platform, waiting with our ticket in hand.

Everything that I have done for Nan is leading to her final journey. I have wrapped each memory tenderly in love before placing it neatly in the case that she will take with her. She will be traveling light, so unburdened by fear that the treasures of this lifetime will have the weight of a feather. And when the time comes and her train is called on some distant platform, I will be there to wish her safe travel and tell her that I will be following her one day. She will smile and turn from me, distracted by the familiar faces pressed against the train windows: her mother, her father, and old friends, all crying her name and waving her aboard. And as the whistle blows she will give me one last glance, then without hesitation she will slowly climb aboard, until all I can see is the shadow of her figure against the closing steel door. And there I will stand, frozen in grief as her car rolls slowly forward, until the cloud of steam becomes so thick that the train vanishes before my eyes, like the flame of an extinguished candle.

EPILOGUE

During the course of writing this book, my sweet Nan passed away at the age of ninety-two. She had a stroke on what seemed like an ordinary Wednesday evening. She had been in high spirits when she and I shared her last supper. But at nine o'clock I received a call explaining that there was a change in her demeanor and that I had best come at once. It was I who accompanied her to the hospital because as is the way of all crises, my husband was out of town on business. In the end nothing could be done to save her since she was left incapacitated and unable to swallow. All we could do was administer palliative care to ensure that her passing was as comfortable as possible. She passed away one month later surrounded by love and in the peaceful setting of our local hospice house.

The final months of 2013 were an especially difficult time for me. Three months before I lost Nan I was diagnosed with non-Hodgkin's lymphoma that required me to have surgery and numerous rounds of chemotherapy. Consequently, in her final days, I was unable to spend a great deal of time with my Nan. As a result of the chemotherapy drugs my immune system was compromised, which made it unwise for me to spend time in hospitals and medical facilities. It may seem odd to say this, but somehow I know that she understood. When I was able to visit she would look at me through bright clear eyes as if she knew exactly what was happening to her—and to me. During my last visit I told her I loved her and that I would look after all those whom she was leaving behind. She nodded and mouthed the words *thank you.*

Cancer has a way of bringing your entire life into sharp focus. It breaks you, shattering all pretenses of promised tomorrows. Before I got sick my life read like an epic poem with endless stanzas stretching far in the future. But now my priorities are recalibrated, honed down into the simplest of poetry, a haiku consisting of seventeen crisp syllables that define my life. Never have I felt more alive. Never have I felt such urgency.

The lessons that I learned from Nan and the times we shared together are precious to me. I can still sense her near me when I feel an unexpected swell of joy or watch a thunderstorm through a dripping wet pane of glass. She is with me when I see clotheslines, unscrew a mason jar, or pass her old market sign as I enter my home. Nan is alive in the trees and in the call of the birds. She is with me when I eat a hot Big Boy tomato right off the vine. I hear her voice in the hymns that I hum while doing my chores. I smell her fragrance in the first lilacs of spring. And when I lay my head down on my pillow at night, she enters my dreams standing on the back porch of her beloved farm. I call to her from down a lane tangled with honeysuckle and Queen Anne's lace until she sees me and waves hello, beckoning me to join her inside. And when I awake, I am still running toward her, heart pounding, trying to reach her before she closes the screen door.

And I am grateful. Grateful for Nan's voice that still rings in my ears. Grateful for her face that smiles down upon me from above. Grateful for all those who I know gathered with open arms to welcome her home.

Godspeed.

NOTES

PROLOGUE

1. Rebecca Mead, "The Sense of an Ending," *The New Yorker* (May 20, 2013), accessed June 5, 2014, http://www.newyorker.com/reporting/2013/05/20/130520fa_fact_mead?currentPage=all.

1. GRABBING AT SHADOWS

1. Alzheimer's Association, "Alzheimer's Facts and Figures," accessed June 5, 2014. http://www.alz.org/alzheimers_disease_facts_and_figures.asp.
2. "Know the 10 Signs," Alzheimer's Association, accessed June 5, 2014. http://www.alz.org/alzheimers_disease_know_the_10_signs.asp.

2. ACCEPTANCE

1. Elisabeth Kübler-Ross, *On Death and Dying* (Scribner Publishing Co., 2011), Kindle edition.
2. Kübler-Ross, *On Death and Dying*.

3. THE MOMENT BY MOMENT TECHNIQUE

1. Viktor E. Frankl, *Man's Search for Meaning* (Beacon Press, 2006), Kindle edition.
2. Thornton Wilder, *Our Town* (Harper Perennial, 2014), Kindle edition.

4. THE JOY CONTINUUM

1. Birgitte Schoenmakers, Frank Buntinx, and Jan Delepeleire, "Factors Determining the Impact of Care-Giving on Caregivers of Elderly Patients with Dementia," *Maturitas* 66 (2010): 191–200, accessed June 20, 2013. doi: 10.1016/j.maturitas.2010.02.09.
2. Esther Oh, MD, "A Case of Depression in a Patient with Dementia" [educational module for Johns Hopkins Geriatric Education Center], 2006. http://www.hopkinsmedicine.org/gec/studies/depression_dementia.html.
3. Oh, "A Case of Depression in a Patient with Dementia."

5. A POSITIVE APPROACH

1. Goodreads, "Dwight D. Eisenhower Quotes," accessed November 2014. http://www.goodreads.com/quotes/128741-pull-the-string-and-it-will-follow-wherever-you-wish.

7. BEAUTY

1. A. J. Lewy, J. I. Numberger, T. A. Wehr, D. Pack, L. E. Becker, and R. L. Powell, "Supersensitivity to Light: Possible Trait Marker to Manic-Depressive Illness," *American Journal of Psychiatry* 142, no. 6 (1985): 725–727.
2. P. D. Sloane, C. M. Mitchell, J. Preisser, C. Phillips, C. Commander, and E. Burke, "Environmental Correlates of Resident Agitation in Alzheimer's Disease Special Care Units," *Journal of the American Geriatrics Society* 46, no. 7 (1998): 862–869.
3. M. E. Copeland and M. McKay, *The Depression Workbook* (California, New Harbinger Publications, Inc., 1992).
4. Kendra Cherry, "Color Psychology," accessed August 13, 2013. http://psychology.about.com/od/sensationandperception/a/colorpsych.htm.

5. Cherry, "Color Psychology."
6. Cherry, "Color Psychology."

8. CREATING EMOTIONAL MEMORIES

1. Meetville, "Quotes and Sayings of Geeta Masurekar," accessed December 29, 2014. http://meetville.com/quotes/quote/geeta-masurekar/64924.

2. William Shakespeare, "Hamlet," In *The Complete Works of William Shakespeare* (London: Oxford University Press, 1963), 886.

3. Rebecca Mead, "The Sense of an Ending," *The New Yorker* (2013), accessed June 5, 2014. http://www.newyorker.com/reporting/2013/05/20/130520fa_fact_mead?currentPage=all.

9. NATURE

1. R. S. Ulrich, "Natural Versus Urban Scenes: Some Psychophysiological Effects," *Environmental Behavior* 13, no. 5 (1981): 523–556. doi: 10.1177/0013916581135001.

2. M. D. Velarde, G. Fry, and M. Tveit, "Health Effects of Viewing Landscapes—Landscape Types in Environmental Psychology," *Urban Forestry & Urban Greening* 6 (2007): 200.

3. Margaret Pickston, *The Language of Flowers* (London: Penguin Group, 1968).

10. THE FIVE SENSES

1. The Quotations Page, "Quotations by Author William Congreve," accessed November 22, 2014. http://www.quotationspage.com/quotes/William_Congreve.

11. MIND GAMES

1. "Activities for People with Alzheimer's Disease," AARP, last modified 2007, accessed June 6, 2014. http://assets.aarp.org/external_sites/caregiving/homeCare/engaging_activities.html.

2. Benjamin P. Sobel, "Bingo vs. Physical Intervention in Stimulating Short-Term Cognition in Alzheimer's Disease Patients," *American Journal Alzheimer's Disease and Other Dementias* 16, no. 2 (2001): 115.

3. "Brain Function: Arithmetic," Brain Center America. http://www.braincenteramerica.com/arithme.php.

4. Henry Ward Beecher, *Proverbs from Plymouth Pulpit* (D. Appleton, 1887), 229.

12. COMMUNICATION

1. Clare Lyons, "Emily Crowhurst Couldn't Have Been Happier," *BBC News Online Network* (1999), accessed October 4, 2013. http://news.bbc.co.uk/2/hi/uk_news/346879.stm.

2. Steven H. Zarit and Judy M. Zarit, *Mental Disorders in Older Adults*, 2nd ed. (Guilford Press, 2001), Google Books edition.

13. DIGNITY

1. Karina Martinez-Carter, "How the Elderly Are Treated around the World," *The Week* (July 23, 2013), accessed August 13, 2013. http://theweek.com/article/index/246810/how-the-elderly-are-treated-around-the-world#axzz33yB2gAJ0.

2. *Holy Bible*, "New International Version" (Grand Rapids, MI: Zondervan, 2011), Luke 10:25–37.

14. SPIRIT

1. "Amazing Grace," *Baptist Hymnal* (Nashville: Convention Press, 1975), No. 165.

2. Zitkala-Sa [Gertrude Simmons Bonnin], *American Indian Stories* (Washington, DC: Hayworth Publishing House, 1921), 101, 107.

16. HUMOR IS THE BEST MEDICINE

1. "Laughter Is the Best Medicine: The Health Benefits of Humor and Laughter," Helpguide.org, accessed April 17, 2014. http://www.helpguide.org/life/humor_laughter_health.htm.

2. Quotery, "Mark Twain Quotes," accessed November 23, 2014. http://www.quotery.com/the-human-race-has-only-one-really-effective-weapon-and/.

17. THE CAREGIVER

1. "Fact Sheet: Selected Caregiver Statistics," accessed October 12, 2013. https://caregiver.org/about-fca.

2. "Fact Sheet: Selected Caregiver Statistics."

3. Maud Purcell, LCSW, CEAP, "The Health Benefits of Journaling," Psych Central, 2013, accessed July 20, 2013. http://psychcentral.com/lib/the-health-benefits-of-journaling/000721.

19. GOING HOME

1. Frank Delaney, *Legends of the Celts* (New York: Sterling Publishing Co., Inc., 1989), 85–96.